CW01023076

The Red F
Revolution

By

Ben Hunt

with

Jeremy Ayres, Phil Escott, Graeme Norbury

OMG.... so good to read! Written so well, and covers so many areas, truth after truth.
Philippa

The best read of the year which will help you to understand how and why you should change your view on the proper human diet and live a full healthier life.
Lidia

Once I started I couldn't stop! It all made so much sense and having followed the advice for the past few months I can say that what Ben and the other authors advocate is absolutely spot on with regards to health and wellbeing. Well researched and not afraid to challenge the narrative that has led us to the diseased societies we find ourselves in. This book should be read by as many people as possible and the knowledge then passed on to future generations.
Emily

Thanks to trying (and failing at) every diet known to man, I thought I was aware of most of the nonsense we've been taught about food. I was so wrong. The Red Pill Food Revolution took me to a whole new level. This will open your eyes to how and, importantly, why we've become sicker and fatter than ever.
Karen

A refreshingly realistic, methodical and logical book on how we've got to where we are. It is clear, a lot of research was put into this. Thoroughly enjoyed listening to it and getting a better grounding on the true reality, rather than the typical narrative of today!! Consolidates a lot of what I believed, with even more insights, that make so much sense. Thank you!
Heather

Spells out in simple terms where we are, what has gone wrong and sets us on a better path for the future.
John

OMG.... so good to read! Written so well, and covers so many areas, truth after truth.
Philippa

The best read of the year which will help you to understand how and why you should change your view on the proper human diet and live a full healthier life.
Lidia

Once I started I couldn't stop! It all made so much sense and having followed the advice for the past few months I can say that what Ben and the other authors advocate is absolutely spot on with regards to health and wellbeing. Well researched and not afraid to challenge the narrative that has led us to the diseased societies we find ourselves in. This book should be read by as many people as possible and the knowledge then passed on to future generations.
Emily

Thanks to trying (and failing at) every diet known to man, I thought I was aware of most of the nonsense we've been taught about food. I was so wrong. The Red Pill Food Revolution took me to a whole new level. This will open your eyes to how and, importantly, why we've become sicker and fatter than ever.
Karen

A refreshingly realistic, methodical and logical book on how we've got to where we are. It is clear, a lot of research was put into this. Thoroughly enjoyed listening to it and getting a better grounding on the true reality, rather than the typical narrative of today!! Consolidates a lot of what I believed, with even more insights, that make so much sense. Thank you!
Heather

Spells out in simple terms where we are, what has gone wrong and sets us on a better path for the future.
John

Chapter 1:
Introduction

We humans are the only creatures in existence that worry and argue about what to eat. Have you ever wondered why that should be?

Something else that makes us unique is the way the vast majority of us live out our lives under a cloud of constant mental and spiritual stress, profoundly dissatisfied and yearning for something different. Is that the way we are meant to live?

Furthermore, although we are told that today's generations enjoy the highest standards of science and healthcare ever known, yet we are getting fatter and sicker, with most of us now doomed to die from a chronic, non-communicable disease for the first time in history. How can we have gotten healthcare so wrong?

Yet another question is, could all these issues somehow be related?

The Red Pill Food Revolution aims to resolve each of those questions and many more, and along the way will expose an incredibly complex illusion of misinformation that has been deliberately crafted in order to disconnect us from our true relationship with our food, with the natural world, and even, as a consequence, with our own spirit.

As you read this book, you will discover something incredibly profound: that food is not only necessary for life, *it is life*. Every animal on Earth knows instinctively what it is meant to do. It spends its time searching out nutrients and energy in the hope that it can survive to procreate and thereby ensure the continued survival of its genes. That quest gives a creature its purpose and its meaning; it is what defines it as a species, unique yet interdependent, only understandable in the context of its complex relationships to the rest of creation.

And then we get to human beings. Supposedly the most intelligent species ever to walk the Earth, humans have somehow forgotten the most fundamental secret to life: what it means to *be* that species. But, as you will learn, somewhere along the way we have not only lost the intrinsic knowledge of what to eat and how to maintain full, vibrant health, but we have also lost touch with what it takes to lead a fulfilling day-to-day existence. We have forgotten our divine birthright... how to be happy.

As you are about to find out in the following chapters, this multi-pronged degeneration all happened within approximately the past fifteen thousand years that follow the end of the Paleolithic Era, a time which witnessed the invention of writing, the creation of money, and which also happens to be the same period that we have been farming the land.

The Red Pill Food Revolution asserts that these parallels are far from coincidences, but rather that the shift from hunting and gathering to agriculture brought with it a radical rupture from nature's laws that triggered a catastrophic cascade of degeneration. Human culture shifted fundamentally away from nature's tendency to universal balance and enrichment and sought to supplant it with an alternative, artificial system that promotes the opposite: imbalance and the enrichment of a few at the expense of the vast majority of people, as well as of the natural world that supports us.

The chapters that follow will take you on a journey all the way from a time before recorded history right up to the present day and, using a combination of science, common sense, and imagination, will illustrate clearly the forces that have caused our precipitous decline.

We will reveal the path that brought our species to this nightmarish existence where we try to exist in two worlds simultaneously: the world of nature, which is real and where every living thing is bound together by universal natural laws into a complex and intricate web of life; and the world of Men, what we call "The System", which foolishly and quite falsely pretends that nature's laws no longer apply.

We will then explore what chance there may be for humanity to save itself from impending collapse, and what each of us can do to help bring that about.

By the end of this journey, you will no longer be confused either about what to eat or why we experience such widespread and deep spiritual malaise with trying to fit into the modern world. You will gain a new appreciation for the profound and mystical place of food at the center of life, how its manipulation over the past few centuries led inevitably to such a sudden and shocking demise in the human condition, and also how we can reverse it.

Along the way you will doubtless experience several shocking revelations, not only about the rapid and accelerating collapse of humanity over recent years, but also about what may be about to happen to us next. We make no apology for that, because if the picture we paint is accurate, it should frankly scare the living daylights out of each one of us. But if that is what it takes for each of us to step up and take action for the sake of our health, our peace-of-mind, our very sense of who we are, and not just for ourselves but for the generations that follow, then we believe it is a pill worth swallowing.

Chapter 2:
How We Are Designed to Eat

To begin solving the puzzle of why we are the only living things that are confused about what we should be eating, we must first get clear about the facts of our natural, species-appropriate food. These facts are absolutely clear to read from our history.

It stands to reason that humans would always have done what every other animal does and learned by copying what our parents or family group ate. It therefore makes sense that *the food that humans have always eaten* must surely be good, healthy, and safe for us.

So what have we *always* eaten?

To understand the human being's natural relationship with food, we have to look at how we have been shaped by the changes in our environment. There is no question that, when it comes to diet, we are extremely adaptable. Both biology and history show that we *can* eat a very wide range of things. (But history also reveals that we have not necessarily always thrived, and that has never been more true than in the past few generations.)

The following chapters will take you on a trip through the history of humanity, *as it is generally understood by science*, to discover how changes in location, environment, technology, and culture have profoundly impacted our food and our health.

Our journey begins in Eastern Africa somewhere around three million years ago. At this time, the Earth was going through the most recent ice age, which locked up a large amount of fresh water in glaciers and consequently caused the climate in tropical regions to become drier.

The rainforests that had previously covered most of the continent gave way to more open spaces, and some groups of the jungle-living apes were forced to leave their dwindling patches of forest and to look for new food sources out on the savannah.

One of these was a small primate that archaeologists call Australopithecus. Fossil records show this little ape stood less than four feet tall, walked upright, and was omnivorous, probably eating mostly fruit along with anything else it might forage like tubers, nuts, and perhaps the occasional lizard.

However out on the grasslands Australopithecus discovered a far richer food source, one which paleontologists believe triggered a remarkable evolutionary transformation.

Recent archaeological discoveries have revealed that Australopithecus was the first ape to use crude stone tools, and also that their hands seem to have adapted to tool use, developing a longer thumb and shorter fingers than other apes. Evidence of cutting marks on bones from the same period show that at some point they also began to butcher meat, which they most likely scavenged from the kills of large predators.

If you observe the behavior of large predators in Africa today, you will see that they always prefer to consume the most nutrient-dense parts of their prey first, which are the internal organs and the fat. Only if they have more time, without being chased off by scavengers like hyenas, will they then move on to eating the muscle meat. It is unlikely that they could get into the largest bones, which contain highly nutritious marrow, or into the skull cavities of their prey and the equally valuable fatty brain tissue locked inside.

However the ability to pick up rocks and smash into bones enabled Australopithecus to access those extra nutrients that were not available to other predators or scavengers. That new source of nutrition triggered a rapid change in physiology. Fossil records reveal that they started to develop larger brains than other primates. For the previous three-and-a-half million years, Australopithecus's brain size had remained constant, but then it quadrupled in size over a relatively short period of time.

That leap in brain capacity can only be explained by a huge increase in the availability of certain key nutrients. Something in the contents of those bony cavities accelerated its evolution, which most scientists believe then progressed swiftly over the next half-million years to the emergence of the genus *Homo* (around two million years ago)... and from there eventually to our species, *Homo sapiens*, somewhere around three hundred thousand years ago according to currently accepted science.

Animals' brains are built mainly out of fats, around sixty percent, as well as a significant amount of cholesterol. In fact a quarter of *all* the cholesterol in your body is found in your brain.

The specific types of fats, or fatty acids, that provide the building material for your brain provide telling clues as to what our early ancestors must have eaten. To grow and to maintain healthy brain tissue, animals need a proper supply of fatty acids, two of which are the omega-3 fatty acids EPA (eicosapentaenoic acid) and DHA (docosahexaenoic acid).

There are dozens of naturally-occurring fatty acids. They all follow a similar pattern, featuring a carboxyl group that is joined to a chain of carbon ions connected to each other and to hydrogen ions. Fatty acids can be categorized by the length of that chain of carbon ions, which range from the shortest having four carbons to the longest with twenty-eight.

EPA is a 20-carbon fatty acid. DHA has a 22-carbon chain. The key point is that DHA is not found anywhere in the plant kingdom, and EPA is present only in trace amounts in some seeds. (It is possible to extract both from certain marine algae.)

In zoology there are two main models of nutrition: there are those animals that eat plants; and there are others that eat the animals that eat plants.

Herbivores—animals that generally eat only plants—get some of the resources their bodies need directly from their food. But they also have the ability to *synthesize* the rest, including the EPA and DHA their brains require.

Carnivores and omnivores either do not have the ability to synthesize these fatty acids, or only a limited ability, but that is not a problem because they can get the nutrients they need by eating other animals. Humans have only a very limited ability to synthesize them from food, via a precursor called ALA (the 18-carbon alpha-linolenic acid).

For that reason, in human nutrition EPA and DHA are termed *essential fatty acids*. The word "essential" refers to the fact that we must get them from our diet. In other words we must conclude that, in order to evolve from Australopithecus to Homo, we *must* have become primarily carnivorous.

Being able to hunt and access more and better nutrients enabled us to continue to grow taller, stronger, and—in particular—smarter. In fact, being able to get more food through hunting large prey with weapons, developing better tools, and cooking with fire has allowed humans to develop *extraordinarily* large brains compared to the size of our bodies. However, carrying an enormous brain had to come at a cost.

In the 1930s, the biologist Max Kleiber observed a pattern common to the vast majority of animals: their metabolic rate, the amount of energy they consumed and expended, was highly predictable. The larger an animal was, proportionally the less energy it needed, so a mouse needs more energy relative to its size than a tiger. However the overall energy needs were close to constant when compared to other animals of a similar mass, and this includes all hominids.

Using Kleiber's Law we can predict accurately the overall amount of energy any animal requires. However the relative proportion of that overall energy budget used by its various organs and muscles may vary. We know that some organs require far more calories than others, in particular the digestive system and the brain.

Anthropologists have shown that, as our early ancestors' brains grew much larger, their guts correspondingly shrank in size, and there is a good reason for this. Brains require a huge amount of energy, and the bigger the brain, the bigger the energy bills.

While your human brain might account for only two percent of your body weight, it uses almost twenty-five percent of your energy, that's nine times more than the rest of the body pound-for-pound. But in order to afford the calories required to run those big brains we were forced to make energy savings elsewhere.

In all other primates, the gut and the liver each use about forty percent of all organ energy usage, amounting to eighty percent in total, with the brain only accounting for around ten percent.

In humans, however, the brain requires *three times more energy*—thirty percent of all organ calorie usage, twenty percent of all your body's energy usage at rest—and the amount of energy used by our gut drops significantly from the forty percent we see in other primates to just twenty-five percent. We are also physically much weaker than other primates, again to make calorie savings to run our brains.

7

Humans have by far the biggest brain, relative to our size, of any large animal. In developing such a massive think box, we did not break Kleiber's Law, but we pushed its boundaries into territories never explored before!

The *expensive tissue hypothesis* explains why, over time, our large intestines had to shrink compared to those of other apes, freeing up energy and allowing our calorie-hungry brains to keep growing. That dramatic reduction in gut size also indicates that our diet must have changed significantly.

Like Australopithecus, almost all other primates had always been predominantly plant eaters, and large herbivorous animals need extensive digestive systems to house the trillions of bacteria that are required to break down plant matter, which the host cannot *directly* digest, into other compounds such as the essential amino acids and fatty acids, which they can.

Herbivorous animals have evolved a variety of large and complex digestive systems, which fall into two main types. Ruminants like cows and sheep have rumens, which start the process of microbial fermentation before the vegetation proceeds to the stomach. These are therefore known as foregut digesters.

Other herbivores, the hindgut digesters, instead have voluminous large intestines and cecums that house the bacteria that do the work of breaking down the plant matter.

Whatever the process, it is interesting to note that even a cow (a ruminant) or an orangutan (a hindgut digester) actually derive most of their energy from short-chain fatty acids. It is a surprising fact that every large mammal actually lives on a high-fat diet, with approximately two thirds or more of their energy coming from those saturated short-chain fatty acids!

Carnivorous animals, on the other hand, tend to have much shorter digestive systems, because the more concentrated and bioavailable nutrients in the meat and fat they consume are quickly broken down into digestible components by the stronger acid and enzymes in the stomach, and can therefore be absorbed more readily, primarily in the small intestine. Note that, like herbivores, carnivores also get at least two thirds of their energy requirements from fatty acids.

Carnivores also do not require large cecums: a digestive component used for bacterial fermentation that sits at the end of the small intestine. A gorilla's cecum is several feet long. In humans the cecum has shrunk right down to the size of your little finger, becoming what we call the appendix.

Note that we do still have billions of bacteria in our gut, and they are extremely important, but they are far too few in number to provide a fraction of our fatty acid requirements from digested plant matter.

Our Unique Dietary Physiology

So we know that humans (Homo) have always been what is known as *facultative carnivores*, which basically means that, while we can eat some plants, we cannot extract all the vital nutrients that our bodies need from the kingdoms of plants and fungi alone. In other words, we are *designed* to get some of the nutrition we need from animal sources.

Having evolved from an omnivorous ancestor means we are able to survive without meat and fat for a period of time, but cannot sustain optimal health long-term that way. However it also means that we differ from other carnivores in a few key aspects. In fact, the natural human diet, which made us human and allowed us to thrive as we colonized most of the world, is unique among animals.

One major difference between us and other carnivores is that, while they are able to break protein down into energy efficiently, humans have never had that ability. While we do have processes to convert some protein into glucose (through a form of gluconeogenesis), this tends to be reserved for times of starvation, allowing us to consume our bodies' own muscle to keep the brain running.

Our current understanding of paleontology points to the fact that, while our very distant ancestors *were* certainly predominantly plant eaters, our brains could only have grown larger and our guts correspondingly smaller in line with the evolution of our diet toward being primarily carnivorous.

Another clue can be found by looking at the *size* of the prey we preferred to hunt. While other apes such as chimpanzees will sometimes hunt in groups to get additional protein, no other ape will attempt to take on an animal that is larger than itself. The only animals that kill larger prey are *hyper-carnivore* predators, defined as those that source at least seventy percent of their food

9

from meat. In that aspect, it could be argued that humans belong in the hyper-carnivore group, sitting at the very "top" of the food chain.

What's more, when researchers used stable isotope analysis to compare the remains of Paleolithic humans to those of other animals, they found an extremely high concentration of certain nitrogen isotopes in the human bones, even compared with other carnivores from the same period. That suggests that we not only hunted herbivorous prey, but sometimes even other carnivores too!

(We must acknowledge that not everybody agrees with the commonly-accepted Darwinian science, which claims that species can not only evolve over time through changes driven by genetic mutation and natural selection, but can also evolve into *new species*. But, however you believe we were designed, whether by evolution, by our environment, by God, or any other means, there is no questioning the numerous facts of our physiology that clearly show *we are designed to eat meat*.)

One example can be seen in the distribution of our fat cells. Omnivores, including the other primates, have a relatively small number of large fat cells, whereas humans' bodies, like those of other carnivores, have a greater number of smaller fat cells.

Also, a human's stomach acid is not only highly acidic, which is typical of carnivores, but it is in fact *even stronger* than that of most other predators, which points to our previous time as scavengers. That's because a scavenger's super-acidic stomach is their critical first line of defense against potentially harmful bacteria that might be present in partly-decayed food. Fierce stomach acid would also have been a benefit later as we hunted much larger prey, which we would have consumed over a period of several days.

As previously mentioned, the rest of our digestive system tells a similar story. Like other carnivores, we have a relatively long small intestine, which is where most of the nutrients in our food are absorbed, but we have a much shorter large intestine than all the other mainly herbivorous primates.

If you observe the shape of a gorilla, for example, you will notice it carries an enormous gut because gorillas are hindgut digesters. Their extensive large intestines are required to house the massive colonies of bacteria that can break down plant matter such as cellulose into the essential nutrients that the gorilla can actually digest and use to fuel, build, and repair their bodies. Because the microbial digestion process is slow and energy-intensive, animals like gorillas must spend the vast majority of every day eating and resting.

If humans ever had the ability to break cellulose down into digestible fatty acids, we must have lost that ability long ago, along with our large, energy-expensive guts. We simply could not power our giant brains at the same time. That means human beings must get the energy we need for day-to-day living from just two remaining macronutrients: fat or simpler carbohydrates.

As humans have small, carnivore-like digestive systems, and because we do not spend most of our time eating as the gorilla does, it stands to reason that our primary source of calories must have come in an energy-dense form.

Carbohydrates, which we might get from starchy plants like tubers or grains, or from the sugars found in fruit, provide four calories of energy per gram, which makes carbs a useful survival food source. But humans found they had access to a far better source of energy and nourishment: fat!

Fat delivers more than twice as much energy as carbs: nine calories per gram. It made sense for our ancestors to expend their energy as wisely as possible to secure the best food sources available. What's more, fat is not only more calorie-rich, but is also far more nutritious.

While carbohydrate-rich plant foods provide energy together with some vitamins and minerals, animal fat contains a much broader spectrum of essential nutrients, including the fat-soluble vitamins A, D, E, and K.

Understanding that animal fat has always been our primary fuel explains why early humans not only preferred to hunt game than to gather tubers, but also why we chose to go for the largest prey animals we could. One simple reason is that larger animals have proportionally greater fat stores than smaller ones.

You can easily see this for yourself in the grocery store. Beef and lamb are clearly far fattier than chicken and rabbit. What is the fattest animal of all, by percentage of body mass? It's the blue whale, also the largest animal that ever existed.

Archeology also provides plenty of evidence pointing to the fact that humans depended on hunting. Not only can we still see ancient cave paintings that exclusively depict hunting scenes, but also the evidence of tools and weapons for use in hunting and for preparing meat goes back much farther than that of tools developed later for processing plant-derived foods.

In addition, at many of the sites in Africa where some of the earliest hominid fossils have been found, large numbers of animal bones were also present. Furthermore, fossilized human feces have been found containing fish bones, fish heads, and feathers but no evidence of preserved seeds or other plant matter.

We now know the facts of our design. Humans are not only adapted to eating animals, but it is actually animal fat in particular that fuelled our incredible growth in intelligence, and with it the power to control our environment. We must conclude that we are designed to eat fatty meat. It contains everything your body needs, and nothing it doesn't.

Chapter 3:
Fat For Life

At this point, you may be experiencing feelings of shock or disbelief at the idea that fat from animals is positive for our health. It is an understandable reaction. After all, we have all grown up *knowing* that, in order to be fit, trim, and healthy, we should strictly limit the amount of saturated fats in our diet. It's just something everyone knows!

In this chapter, we will present you with further unequivocal proof that fat is not only *not* the health risk that you have been told it is, but that quite the opposite is true! Animal fat is *absolutely essential to human health.*

The question as to *why* we have been raised in the certain knowledge that saturated fat is a killer is actually of critical importance, and the search for an answer is at the core of this book, so it will become clear as you read on.

As we have stated before, common sense dictates that the proper diet for any species is *the food that species has always eaten.* For example, lions have *always* eaten warm-blooded herbivores, orcas have *always* eaten fish and seals, moles have *always* eaten earthworms, rabbits have *always* eaten grass, while rats have *always* eaten a wide range of foods.

Because we know that humans managed to thrive and to occupy most of the land on Earth during the last ice age, we can say that, like rats, *what we've always eaten* includes a wide range of foods, but we can also see conclusive evidence that it must always have included significant quantities of fatty meat or fish.

First, the fact that dietary animal fats are essential to long-term survival is clear from a quick look into anthropology, because they form part of the diet of every known indigenous population.

A Corrected Ethnographic Atlas, published in 1999, was a survey of around two hundred and forty still-existing indigenous tribes. It found that seventy-three percent of those tribes got at least half of their food from animal sources. The two tribes that

13

ate the most plant foods still derive six and fifteen percent of their diet from animal sources respectively. There was not a single indigenous tribe found living anywhere on Earth today that abstains from foods from animals.

Here is a selection of examples of what some of those indigenous tribes eat:

• The Maasai of Tanzania and Kenya thrive almost exclusively on the blood, milk, and meat from their cattle. They are also famed for their exceptional health and athletic ability.

• The Hadza, who also live in Tanzania, prefer meat, and also eat some plants. When they do eat starchy tubers, they will chew on them and then spit out the indigestible fiber.

• The Sámi reindeer herders of Northern Europe thrive almost exclusively on the milk and meat of their reindeer.

• The Inuit of Northern Canada live on fatty seal and whale meat and fish, again almost exclusively.

• The Tukisenta of Papua New Guinea have probably the lowest proportion of diet from animal sources, getting as many as ninety-five percent of their calories from a wide variety of yams (sweet potatoes), which they supplement with oily fish from the sea. The Tukisenta are generally very healthy but can be prone to diabetes, which is extremely rare among indigenous peoples who continue to eat their ancestral diet. (Also note that yams only reached Papuya New Guinea in the last five hundred years.)

In fact the idea of humans surviving without food from animal sources at all is a very recent phenomenon.

So we can say with confidence that, all along our journey from the African plains to every corner of the Earth, animal meat and fat have *always* been the mainstay of humans' diets. In some areas, we might supplement with other available food sources, but we must conclude that—excluding a small minority in very recent times—*the only food that humans have always eaten is flesh and fat.*

Therefore common sense dictates that flesh and fat *must* be our most natural and most health-enhancing food. This is also backed up by yet more solid evidence from human biology.

In fact, really you do not have to look any further than one of the main topics of the previous chapter: our big brains.

We have already seen how humans could *only* have developed our unusually massive brains thanks to a diet that was high in animal fats, as they provide the only rich enough source of 20- and 22-carbon fatty acids (EPA and DHA) that our brains need to grow.

Now you might argue that, while we *may* have needed all that fat from eating brains and bone marrow in order to evolve originally into the Homo genus, perhaps we have since continued to evolve again to the point where we no longer need to consume animal fats.

But this is clearly not the case. The fact remains that we still all need a sufficient amount of those essential fatty acids in our diets today in order to maintain our brains.

A study published in 2008 presented the results of an experiment that tracked the changes in brain size, measured using brain scans, in over a hundred individuals aged between 61 and 87, over a five year period. While the focus of the study was to investigate the importance of vitamin B12 in brain deterioration, it also threw up some startling discoveries.

When correlating the subjects' diets with changes in brain mass, the scientists discovered that those who ate no meat were six times more likely to suffer brain shrinkage, and the vegans in the study (those who abstain from all animal products, even dairy and eggs) experienced the most shrinkage of all, losing on average more than five percent of their total brain mass in just five years.

What's more, when the subjects were scanned at the start of the trial, the largest brain belonging to a vegan subject measured 1455cc in volume, whereas the *smallest* brain from a non-vegan was 1456cc. So every single one of the vegans had a smaller brain volume than all of the omnivores, and they shrank even more over the period of the study!

This experiment alone points to the fact that getting enough essential fatty acids in the diet is an absolute requirement in order to maintain a full-sized human brain.

We also come to the same conclusion regarding the importance of dietary fat when we recall the fact that *all* large mammals live on a high-fat diet, even those that eat only plants.

As we have seen, aside from getting some energy from starch and sugar, herbivores meet about 70% of their calorie needs from short-chain fatty acids, which in their case they ferment in their digestive systems with the help of vast colonies of symbiotic bacteria.

Carnivores also get about 70-80% of their energy needs from fats, which they get from their prey, herbivores that have already built the essential nutrients with the help of bacteria.

Because human beings do not have the rumens, large cecums, or long large intestines that are required to ferment plant matter into short-chain fatty acids, we simply *cannot* get the crucial fats that we need from bacterial fermentation. We simply don't have the equipment.

That means we can only get the energy we need from two main macronutrient sources: fats and/or carbohydrates. But are they equally good fuel sources?

No, we cannot get all our energy exclusively from carbs and remain healthy in the long term. Carbohydrates provide calories, but that is all. They are fundamentally lacking in numerous other essential nutrients.

The simple reality is that our bodies need far more than just energy; all of our cells need *sufficient nutrition* in order to do the building and repair work required to maintain full health.

Fat and carbohydrates are both natural forms of stored energy. Plants, being simpler organisms, use energy in the form of sugars, so their storage is either simple sugars like glucose and fructose, or starch, which is simply lots of glucose molecules joined together. Because plants are not so limited by size and weight as animals are, they can just grow more and larger stems above ground or more and larger tubers below ground.

However animals have different priorities. Our muscles and liver can store a modest amount of energy in the form of glycogen (up to a maximum of around fifty thousand calories), which is useful in case we need to spring into action urgently. But carbohydrate is not our most efficient long-term storage mechanism, for two main reasons: it is too bulky; and it cannot hold other vital nutrients.

We know that carbohydrates and protein provide four calories of energy per gram, whereas fat stores more than twice that, supplying nine calories per gram. The logical reason is that, because animals have to move around and therefore carry their energy stores with them, nature had to find the most efficient possible solution that offered the maximum calorie-to-weight ratio.

In addition to providing a massive amount of energy, fat also delivers a full range of essential fat-soluble vitamins, which are... Vitamin A, essential for eye and skin health; Vitamin D, which strengthens the immune system, muscles, and bones; Vitamin E, a crucial antioxidant; Vitamin K, required to help your blood to clot; and Vitamin K2, which controls the flow of calcium in the body, bones, teeth, putting it where it's needed and preventing calcification in places where it is not helpful.

But what's more, fat is also *in itself* an essential building block for our bodies. We already know that sixty percent of the dry weight of your brain is made up of fat. But fat also forms part of the membrane of every cell in your body. In addition it functions as a structural component and as essential protection for the organs such as the eyes, liver, lungs, and skin. And of course fat is also a major ingredient in bone marrow, which creates blood cells and stem cells, as well as most of the hormones that your body uses for signaling and regulation.

In other words, fat is quite literally *essential to who you are*!

It stands to reason that, precisely *because* it has been designed to store what an animal needs, animal fat must naturally contain the ideal mix of all the fatty acids along with the fat-soluble vitamins our bodies require, all together in one super-efficient package.

Let's now consider the various reasons *why* animals create fat to store energy and nutrients.

Of course, animals store fat reserves for their own bodies to use as an efficient reserve of calories and vitamins. And body fat also provides vital insulation to land and sea creatures that live in cold regions.

But fat's ability to store energy and nutrition also plays a vital role in animal reproduction, which offers even more evidence of why it *must* be the perfect human fuel.

Birds, reptiles, amphibians, and fish produce eggs, which must contain everything a developing embryo needs to grow to viability in a self-contained package. That's why all eggs are high in fat, not in carbohydrates.

A further source of animal fats found in nature is the larvae of insects and other invertebrates, which must also carry significant energy reserves in the most efficient way, and fat again is nature's best solution.

It is relevant to note that all of these fatty food sources (meat, fish, eggs, and grubs) have always been favored by indigenous peoples. Our ancestors, as well as those tribes that live on the land in the modern era, would have been familiar with *any and all* of these premium sources of energy and nutrition that are available in their part of the world.

Of course there is one more critically important use of fat in the reproductive process, which is the milk of mammals. The mammalian procreation strategy is to grow their young for a period within their bodies and then to provide additional nutrition after birth through suckling on milk.

The macronutrient content of human breast milk again points to how crucial fat must be to our health. And it comes back, yet again, to our big brains.

Human babies are *extraordinarily* fat at birth. In fact they carry more fat than even a newborn gray seal, and for a very important reason.

When fully developed, our brains are so big that a human baby simply could not pass through the birth canal. For that reason, our offspring come out only partly developed. Human babies have much smaller brains compared to their parents than those of other primates, which are born more or less fully-developed.

Human infants' brains must finish building rapidly after birth, including the crucial period sometimes called "the second nine months". While they come out with only half-built brains, they are also provided with many of the materials needed to finish the job. This is in the form of their rolls of body fat, which are stored up during gestation and can also pass through the birth canal safely. This body fat is not only high in all the essential fats, but also in stem cells.

Babies' other vital source of additional nutrition comes of course from their mother's milk, which contains between three and five percent fat, of which almost half is saturated fat, high amounts of DHA, as well as vitamins and nutrients, and some sugar in the form of lactose. Fifty-five percent of the calories a baby gets comes from fat, with a little from protein and the remainder from the sugars.

Let's apply a little common sense again here.

Why would a diet that is very high in saturated fat be ideal for a human baby, but then suddenly become less than optimal, or even a health risk, later in life? What could change so dramatically between the physiology of a human infant and adult?

If, as it is clear to see with your own eyes, human babies are designed to consume a high-fat, in fact a *high-saturated-fat*, diet, it is impossible for that same type of macronutrient mix then to turn toxic in maturity.

If consuming fat made us obese, then babies would get even fatter, not leaner, throughout the nursing period.

If fat made us sick, more babies would suffer ill health and fewer would make it to adulthood.

No, a high-saturated-fat diet cannot logically be ideal during one stage of a human being's life and then life-threateningly dangerous in another.

If further proof should be needed, you only have to consider the fact that humans have always used the same way of storing energy to get through the winter months: our own animal fat! We store fat when energy is more plentiful in our environments, and then break down that fat again to provide energy when food is scarce. How can the exact same fuel source be at once nature's ideal solution for making it through winter when obtained from our own fat cells, but also unhealthy when obtained through consuming the fat of other animals' in our diet?

Therefore a diet high in animal fats has never been, and cannot be, anything less than ideal for human beings.

"But... science!!"

Right now your brain is likely to be fizzing with conflictions. You have seen all the evidence and common sense that point to the conclusion that a high-fat diet must be both natural and healthy, yet on the other hand... *everybody knows* that saturated fats are a health hazard.

And you are almost right... Everybody *is* raised being told to avoid or at least to limit saturated fat in the diet, that vegetable oils are "heart healthy", that we should get more whole grains, and so on. Because of science!

But the fact that *everybody knows* something does not make that thing true. And that is what The Red Pill Food Revolution is all about. We have lost our instinctual knowledge about our natural diet and instead have been sold a pack of lies.

The reality is, *not everybody* knows that saturated fat is bad, despite the constant wall-to-wall propaganda we have grown up with. However, as we will realize as we progress on our journey of discovery, dissenting voices are frequently silenced in favor of the orthodox, mainstream message.

Indeed there have always been outliers who have engaged in real, actual, honest science, and who have seen the truth for themselves. We will meet several of these outliers, these true scientists, as we continue our journey through the ages.

You are going to see two very different pictures emerge. One shows a type of science that is funded by, and totally dependent on, big money and industry. This science is carefully managed so that its findings match the desired outcomes of its sponsors.

The other is the true science, which is pursued by the outliers whose only goal is truth. These pioneers look at the world as it is, with open eyes. They are ready to challenge their preconceptions, opinions, and even all their previous education. If the evidence shows a reality that conflicts with their current beliefs, they are prepared to throw away those beliefs and try on new ones.

As you proceed through this book, we hope you can adopt a similar approach. Be ready to have everything you have been told challenged and, in many cases, completely overturned, particularly as it relates to fat and *all* the information you have been fed so far about healthy eating.

The fat-fuelled human

Finally, let us look at another key feature of human physiology, and what it tells us about our ancestral (and therefore natural) eating habits. Fat is not only our perfect natural fuel, but it also plays a big role in *how* we should eat.

It is interesting to note that humans are significantly fatter than any other primate, and by a staggering margin! For example take the bonobo, the pygmy chimpanzee, which is thought to be genetically our nearest cousin. Female bonobos tend to have around four percent body fat, and the males close to none at all. Other apes have a similarly low body fat percentage.

How much body fat does a healthy human carry? Typically thirty-six percent if you are a woman and twenty percent if you are a man! We are far, far fatter than any of the other apes, even the ones with gigantic bellies!

Why would we need to store so much body fat? Why would nature have made us fat by design?

A gorilla spends about half its day eating, and a significant portion of the remaining time resting (because digestion is hard work). Consider that gorillas live in forests where they are surrounded by food, so they do not need to move much and can simply munch the day away. Plus their environment is also warm, so they have no need for extra insulation. For a gorilla, to carry a load of body fat would simply be unnecessary and inefficient.

There are plenty of other large land animals that do carry far more body fat. A healthy dog, for example, has between fifteen and twenty percent body fat, whereas a lion would carry around thirteen percent.

A human's body fat percentage is closer to that of a Labrador, which is a carnivore, than that of a chimp, which is mainly herbivorous. This would make sense if we have adapted to an eating pattern based on hunting, where we would experience occasional successful kills interspersed by periods of less food.

Just like with all animals, every cell in our bodies needs a steady supply of energy, which as we know must come either from carbohydrates, which are broken down into sugars, or fats, which are broken down into ketones.

A gorilla, a cow, or a rabbit has no trouble getting its steady supply of energy. It spends most of the day moving around slowly and munching on the abundant plant matter, which as we know ferments in its belly, the bacteria breaking it down into the short-chain fatty acids, which the animal then digests and uses to provide constant energy, along with a modest amount of carbohydrate (dead bacteria providing the amino acids it requires to build its body).

Carnivorous predators, such as wolves or leopards or sperm whales, have more sporadic eating patterns and will often go for days on end with no food. That's why carnivores have more fat cells and carry more body fat. They are *designed* to consume their own fat stores between kills.

The reason that carnivores do not need to eat constantly is precisely *due to* the nature of their diet. That's because the mainstay of their fuel supply is fat: energy-dense *animal fats* from their food along with their own stored fat.

Appetite and hunger are primarily driven not by the presence of food in your belly, but by the availability of *energy and nutrition*. Because they are high in both energy and nutrient value, animal fats are extremely satiating, in fact it is very hard to keep eating fat when you have had enough (unlike many other food sources, as we will see later). When you get enough high-quality fat in your diet, you simply do not feel any desire to keep on eating.

Consider that you never actually *stop* eating... you only stop putting stuff in your mouth. Your body is always eating. If it does not get immediately available energy from sugars or ketones in the blood, it will draw that energy from glycogen stores in the liver and pancreas and from fatty acid stores in your fat cells.

When your body has enough energy, from food or from stored fat, *together with enough other nutrients*, again from food or from stored fat, it will be in a happy, optimal state. That means you will also not feel hungry. After all, why would your body cause you discomfort when there is no biological need?

(This realization provides one clue as to why people these days get obese. One reason they overeat is because they *are* genuinely frequently hungry, and the reason they are frequently hungry is because what they are consuming is low in fat and therefore not satiating. So they can eat and eat, but if what they are putting in their mouths delivers only short-term energy without sufficient nutrients, their bodies can never say it's time to stop, but will keep shouting for nutrition.)

The reality is, like other carnivores, you are not designed to eat constantly, rather you are designed to function perfectly well on a sporadic eating pattern. Our ancestors, being primarily hunters, would certainly not have eaten all the time, but would have gorged in times of plenty, just as other predators do, and fasted in the periods between kills as well as over the winter.

With our generous fat stores, humans are designed to thrive with a fairly significant buffer of stored energy, constantly switching between storing and then recycling body fat.

Imagine that the fat cells in your body have one-way doors, which can switch between "entry only" or "exit only". They are always either in storage mode, when they can receive energy, or they are in release mode, gradually delivering that energy back out into the bloodstream for the rest of the cells in the body to use.

When you have had a meal that includes carbohydrates, your blood sugar will rise, triggering production of the hormone insulin, which tells your fat cells to go into storage mode. When in a fasted state, the blood insulin level will drop, which then tells the fat cells to switch into release mode, so that you can carry on going, now using the stored fats (converted to ketones) as fuel.

In fact, far from being a hardship, being able to function in a fasted state between feasts also delivers many significant health benefits.

Although food is of course essential to life, the act of digesting it also puts a level of stress on the body. Any time you consume food, your digestive system must jump into action.

The release of insulin acts as a general alert signal, preparing your body to deal with the incoming food. Aside from telling fat cells to go into storage, another effect is that extra blood will be redirected from your muscles to the digestive system. That's why you can often feel tired and cold after a large meal. Remember, digestion is hard work.

Fasting—periods of time between digestive duties—also gives the body more time to repair itself through a process called autophagy. Autophagy is a vital cell repair mechanism in which old or redundant cells and cellular components get recycled and replaced. Cells are marked for repair when you are awake to be repaired later during the night, as part of a complex and elegant chain of maintenance processes that happen during sleep.

This chain of events, like many other bodily processes, is managed by the timed release of hormones. But the presence of insulin can interrupt that sequence, preventing the full repair cycle from completing during the night.

If our ancestors ate only when food was available, and then most likely only during daylight hours, they would usually have slept in a fasted state, with minimal levels of insulin in the blood, ensuring a fully refreshing and recharging night's sleep. If we are constantly eating, this repair cycle can never fully complete.

A further benefit of the feasting-fasting pattern relates to toxins. One of the many ways your body uses stored fat is to sequester toxins that have entered from the external environment. When your body is in its normal fasted state, it is recycling its stored fat for energy, which also means any toxins are slowly released at a rate that your organs of excretion (the liver, kidneys, skin, lungs, and bowel) can deal with. So a pattern of frequent fasting allows you regularly to expel any undesirable toxic chemicals.

In summary, we have now seen how fat—and specifically fat from animals—was not only our most essential food source throughout human evolution, but that it clearly remains so today, which of course flies in the face of the education we have all been sold. The lessons of our biology seem to contradict the teaching served up by the authorities!

It is possible to understand how we came to find ourselves in this state of profound conflict and confusion about something so simple as how to feed ourselves. We will uncover all the clues we need as we continue our journey through the timeline of human history.

In the next chapter we will immerse ourselves deeper into stone age life in order to understand more intimately not only *what* we ate, but *how* we related to food for the overwhelming majority of our time here on Earth.

Chapter 4:
Ancestral Living

The vast majority of human existence, around ninety-five percent of the entire timespan from when the first humans walked the earth up to the present day, took place in what is known as the Paleolithic period.

Modern humans are still genetically and biologically practically identical to our Paleolithic ancestors, whom we typically think of as cavemen. That means our most natural and species-appropriate way of living and feeding ourselves comes straight out of the stone age. ("Paleo" means "old" and "lith" means "stone".)

Thanks to their huge brains, our ancestors were able to develop technology that allowed them to become the most efficient hunters the world had ever seen. In particular, they invented projectile weapons: the spear; then the spear thrower; and later bows and arrows about 23,000 years ago.

Early man's superior intelligence also led to the invention of language, which enabled our ancestors to hunt even more effectively. Communication is a huge help when hunting in teams, which is why highly intelligent predators like painted dogs and wolves, dolphins and orcas are so lethally efficient.

Those key advances meant primitive human hunters were able to take down large prey of their own and so get all the best nutrients from the organs, fat, and bone marrow as well as all the meat for themselves. They had also harnessed the power of fire, possibly up to 700,000 years ago, which unlocked yet more potential nutrition from their food.

So you could say that hunting, preparing, and cooking *our own food* is the key factor in what made us human, what fundamentally defines us as a species. It is also clear that we were not solitary hunters but lived and hunted in bands, which meant we could tackle the largest and fattest prey animals, the megafauna of the Paleolithic.

It is tempting to assume that, for the entire time humans have existed, the climate has been more or less the same as we observe today, but in fact that is not the case.

According to geologists, around two and a half million years ago the world entered into a cooler phase, caused by regular variations in the Earth's orbit around the sun, and that led to a series of ice ages, interspersed with shorter, warm interglacial periods.

The earliest remains of Homo sapiens found in East Africa appear to be around two hundred thousand years old. It is generally understood that Homo sapiens moved out of Africa to colonize most of the rest of the world between sixty and ninety thousand years ago.

The vast majority of the time humans have been on the Earth was actually dominated by two ice ages, long periods during which the Earth's average temperature dropped so low that large areas were left permanently under thick ice, with glaciers extending over much of the land's surface in northern latitudes, and locking up so much water that the tropics will have been much drier than they are today.

The first ice age started around two hundred thousand years ago and lasted for approximately seventy thousand years. Then followed an interglacial period that lasted about twenty thousand years, then another ice age that ended only eleven thousand years ago, giving way to the temperate interglacial period that we are in right now.

Those ice ages will only have allowed a short potential growing period during the summer, and scientists also believe that, due to colder sea temperatures, the levels of carbon dioxide in the atmosphere were about half of what they are today. The net result is that the land would have supported far less vegetation than we see now, and the plant species that did grow would have to be very hardy.

The types of animals that could have thrived in those cold climates would need to grow as large as possible because having more body mass compared to surface area is more efficient at retaining heat. They would also need to be able to find food such as lichens and mosses under the snow, just as musk oxen, elk, and reindeer do today.

That means our stone age ancestors must surely have relied on hunting large prey to survive in the extended cold conditions, as the majority of prehistoric cave paintings confirm.

So Paleolithic living, and the food that was central to it, provides a benchmark for our understanding of the natural human condition. Since that age came to an end, only around eleven thousand years ago, we have moved a long way from that natural state.

In this chapter we will pay a visit to the Paleolithic as fully appreciating the way we evolved to live will provide the necessary foundation for understanding the key role that food has played in the cause of modern humanity's biggest problems.

Obviously every one of us needs to eat to stay alive and that has not changed. Even today when times are hard we say that our ultimate concern is "putting food on the table". Being able to eat and to provide for our loved ones is still a central priority for everyone.

And food will always continue to be an absolute necessity. However, the food we ate and the way that we relate to it changed dramatically and, on an evolutionary timeline, extremely suddenly. In fact, we will show how it also led to the establishment of new, unequal power structures.

Going far beyond a simple question of survival for our ancestors, food will have been absolutely central to their way of life. Aside from the other basic necessities of shelter, security, and fire, life was *all about food*: learning what is safe and good to eat; planning how to get it; sourcing it; preparing it; being grateful for it; and sharing it.

So we have always had a deep, ancestral, emotional connection with our food, which would have bound us to our natural place in the world. While the food that different people eat can vary from place to place, its importance does not.

But in recent times something radical and deeply worrying has changed around how we relate to food. What was always a source of life, health, connection, and delight has now been corrupted into a weapon that is being used against us.

In order that you can fully appreciate how that could have come about, let us take some time to reconnect with that crucial aspect of our ancestral memory.

That's because how we relate to our food is no trivial thing. In fact it is the key to unlocking many of our most pressing modern problems, not only as it relates to your and your family's physical health, but to our psychological and emotional wellbeing too, and even the future of human life on Earth.

Let's now imagine what life might have been like for humans living towards the end of the prehistoric stone age, starting early one spring morning. (Be sure to note the way each day is primarily structured by the available sunlight at each particular time of year.)

You wake up with the sunrise on a crisp morning and step outside of your shelter. You greet two of the men of the tribe who took the last watch, looking out for potential dangers and keeping the fire going through the night.

Other members of the group emerge and start to discuss the day ahead. You grab a strip of some dried meat that has been hanging in the smoke of the fire to protect it from insects and scavengers.

A party of around twenty men talk strategy as they get ready to go out for the day's hunt. It has been several days since the tribe got a kill, but the herds now have their young, which thankfully means hunting should be relatively easy at this early time of year, although because the days are still short the hunters cannot venture very far.

Everyone looks lean but well rested after the winter. A few of the women have recently given birth, which always gives cause for good cheer around the camp. The tribe's numbers have swelled over the past few years.

A few youngsters go off to collect fresh water from the stream, which they bring back in tanned leather bags, and to check on the fish traps. Someone else heads out to forage for a particular spring moss, which has healing properties and should be growing nearby.

After the sun has peaked and started to creep downwards towards the treeline, the hunters come back to an enthusiastic welcome. They have been lucky! An old elk that made it through the winter was now too slow and made for an easy kill. There are shouts of delight and congratulations all round.

Suddenly the camp is a hive of activity. Everyone quickly gets to work removing every part of the animal using a variety of specialized tools. Organs and meat are removed using flint knives, and a couple of men set about breaking into the elk's limb bones and skull using stone axes.

Absolutely no part of the animal is wasted. The rich organ meats are set aside to cook and eat later that day, and the muscle meat is carefully sliced and hung over the fire. The hide is then scraped clean ready to be dried and then tanned.

As the sky turns orange and red everyone enjoys a good feast. Food is carefully divided so that everyone has enough, with more organs going to anyone who is sick or pregnant. Particular provision is also made for girls approaching childbearing age.

The days are starting to get longer, but night still draws in early at this time of year. As the sky turns darker, you spend a while sitting around the fire with a full belly as some of the hunters recount stories from the day's adventures. One of the elders then tells some of the fables of the tribe's history as the youngsters listen on intently.

There is a short discussion of when it may be the best time to move camp up to the higher plain, as the tribe does every year. A few voices chip in with considerations, and finally a decision is agreed on. As darkness closes around the campfire and you start yawning, it is time to crawl back into your shelter, climb under your skins, and sink into a deep sleep.

The following day everyone rests, only carrying out the light chores that need to be done. Everyone has their own set of skills that help the tribe to thrive. A couple of adults help their neighbor make repairs to their shelter, another casually sits carving a wooden bowl, a few take care of preparing the elk hide, while an older man teaches some of the kids how to knap flint to make arrowheads. The spring air is full of chatter peppered with frequent laughter.

A few months later, the landscape looks transformed. All of nature is in abundance. Up on the high plain the prairie grasses have grown to full height and most have gone to seed. Bushes are heavy with berries and a few nuts are starting to appear on the trees.

Hunting is not quite as easy as it was in the springtime, as this year's young have grown stronger and faster, but the days are long and everyone is bursting with energy so the men can stay out for most of the day and regularly bring a nice, fat animal back to the camp. Now, with meat and forageable food in abundance, everyone is starting to look much plumper, which is a very good sign.

As summer gives way to autumn and the days begin to shorten, everyone starts to turn their attention to the coming winter. Any spare meat is carefully sliced, dried and ground, then combined with fat to make a kind of fatty cake that will keep for a long time and provide crucial sustenance through the cold months ahead.

As winter draws in, everyone carefully checks the stores of supplies, knowing that there may be little opportunity to find fresh food once the snows come. As the days get ever shorter, you feel your body slowing down as it prepares for rest. By now the bears and marmots will already be in their nests underground to sleep out the winter.

Each day during the winter months offers less sunlight, so everyone gradually sleeps longer, coming out only to relieve themselves, share a small meal, gather wood, and get warm by the fire. Some days a hunting party may go out to see what they can find, but the short hours of daylight and harsh conditions mean that the chances of a successful hunt are unpromising.

As each day passes the sun gradually disappears earlier and earlier. This is time to rest, repair, and prepare. Most of the tribe spend the short days around the camp crafting useful things such as tools and arrows, weaving baskets, twisting twine, or working leather into bags and boots.

The campfire chat now turns to the longest night of the winter when the elders always lead a special celebration anticipating the sun's return and looking forward hopefully to another good year. Fortunately, the previous summer was abundant and the tribe has been able to put plenty of provisions aside to see everyone safely through the long, cold winter.

As midwinter approaches, the faces that had been fat and round a few months ago are starting to look a little leaner again, but it won't be too long till spring comes around once more. You feel a deep swell of gratitude rise inside you. Nature has been generous and kind to the tribe once again.

Visualizing life through a complete Paleolithic year in this way helps us start to appreciate how, over countless millennia, human biology has been precisely designed by our environment, by the changing of the seasons, and by whatever sources of nourishment were available. Note that there was no one typical day, and no single way of eating; you would consume whatever nature provided, depending on the season. Everything worked in perfect harmony, all driven primarily by the sun's cycles.

Let's explore in further detail some of the key factors of stone age tribal life, as really getting a feel for how we evolved to live through the vast majority of our existence will be extremely helpful in helping us to understand why and how the human condition has degenerated so much in the modern age.

Food

We'll start with food and the fat storage cycle. When food was plentiful, nothing ever went to waste, and our ancestors would store as much energy as they could in body fat ready for the lean months. That is a very good thing, as it means they were in the happy position to turn the excess available calories into reserves that would help them survive the winter.

If we accept that the way your body works was in some way designed by our Paleolithic ancestry, we could say we *are meant to* get fat during one particular part of the year. We are then *meant to* burn off that extra fat during the winter. On a shorter cycle, we would also store some fat following a successful hunt when there was an abundance of food, and could use that stored energy to keep going until the next kill.

That is how your body is designed to survive in challenging conditions. Storing fat is far from a problem but rather an essential survival strategy! *Being* fat is not a problem; it means you have energy stored to keep you going until you get food again. It was, and is, also crucially important for women to build up sufficient fat reserves before getting pregnant.

In particular, take note of how the diet high in animal fats allowed people not only to survive the winter, but also to go for days on end with no food without suffering distress.

Food was still the central focus of life. It literally *was* life! As long as the other basic needs were taken care of, most of every day's activity would revolve primarily around all the activities involved in food provision.

Closely linked to that central focus on food is the sacred act of giving thanks. As food literally meant life to our ancestors, it was never taken for granted, but always fully appreciated. A successful hunt would be cause for joy and celebration. Every good meal that the tribe shared would instill feelings of profound gratitude: to nature, to the hunters, to those who prepared the food, and of course to the spirit of the animal.

Activity

In a natural ancestral lifestyle there is no distinction between "work" and recreation, rather days would be a mix of times of activity and times of rest. Any activity could be enjoyable, and they would very often be carried out socially.

By definition, because we thrived for millennia off the land, nature must have provided everything we needed. In a natural, ancestral existence anything you might require must be out there for the taking or for the making. If you needed a shelter or a spear or a pair of boots, you would simply go out and get the resources you needed from the natural world.

Activity would also be its own reward. Because of the immediacy of working with the natural resources that are all around, everyone would see and enjoy the results of their labor straight away.

There would also be no distinction of "education". Everyone had their own set of skills and would also constantly be trying out ideas, learning, and teaching others. It made sense for everyone to be keen to know how to do what they could to help the tribe.

When whatever needed to be done was done, there would have been plenty of time for rest and relaxation. Taking care of all your needs required just a few hours of activity most days.

This is still true for today's remaining hunter-gatherers, who get all their needs met typically "working" for only fifteen to twenty hours per week!

No two days would ever be the same. Each individual would be more or less self-directed, doing only what work was required. If nothing needed to be done, you would not do anything.

More significant effort may have been expended when tribes made their frequent migrations, moving camp to be closer to various food sources throughout the year, perhaps following migrating herds or spawning fish.

Harmony

The tribe's use of resources would always be kept in check. While nature does provide in abundance, it simply would not make sense to take more than you needed.

There would be no point in having more spears or hide boots than the tribe could make use of. There was no point killing more animals than you could eat. To over-harvest resources would simply waste time and energy for no additional benefit.

It simply made sense to do what was required to take care of yourself and the tribe and your environment. Everyone benefited when the tribe was strong and healthy. So you would only ever take what you needed.

Taking too much from the natural world could even be a danger to the tribe. If you over-fished a lake, over-hunted a herd, or cut down all the trees, you might jeopardize the future supply of those resources.

The way we consumed was directly and intimately linked to our survival. We had to consume, but at the same time could not take too much, or we would risk suffering shortage in the future. So we lived with a natural tendency toward balance and harmony.

Population

Because of the importance of not harvesting too much from the world around us, tribes would probably have faced a natural size limit, probably in the region of one hundred individuals.

A human being is probably only really able to know and to trust up to one hundred other faces. Consider also that, in a tribe, everyone would want to gather round the campfire in a council, and that would not be workable with a very large group.

A further natural constraint might be the number of people required to take down, cut up, transport, and consume an entire large animal, so that everyone could enjoy their fair share, but without any going to waste.

Too many people might also dilute the integrity of the tribe's hive mind, making it hard to keep track of who was doing what task.

A tribe needed to be large enough to allow for sufficient division of labor, and also redundancy in case some members were heavily pregnant, nursing, or injured.

For these reasons, if a tribe grew too big, it might divide with one group moving off to find new land.

Interdependency

Each tribe's elders would help keep alive its particular oral traditions, the tribal *lore* that reminded everyone of their true place in the world, of the importance of harmony and how to maintain it. Preserving that traditional knowledge was essential to the tribe's integrity and success.

In a natural, intimate, and equitable tribal culture, there would be no occasion for crime, because any benefit would be tiny compared to the risk. Everyone knew everyone, and everyone knew what everyone else was doing most of the time. The security of belonging to a strong tribe was far more important than any fleeting individual gain.

Anyone would of course be free to leave the tribe and to make their own way in the world, but it would not make sense to abandon the benefits of the division of labor and the greater overall protection and edification that the tribe offered.

For that reason, there would be no need for laws. It stands to reason that decisions that affect the tribe should be made around the campfire. Perhaps the campfire council was the original true democracy, which means government by the people, in which everybody could hear what is said and anybody could have a voice.

An idea or action would make sense if it benefited the tribe, and there was really no reason to pursue individual advancement at the cost of anyone else or the group.

It made sense that any resources would be distributed equitably, because the tribe's strength *was* the combined strength of all its members. What benefited an individual benefited the tribe, and what benefited the tribe in turn benefited everyone, resulting in a natural, cyclical system of mutual cooperation.

However, if an individual was unable to coexist harmoniously with the tribe, they would surely not last long but face swift judgment, likely resulting in banishment. Because the integrity and security of the tribe were literally life-or-death issues a tribe might not be able to tolerate an individual who exhibited psychopathic tendencies.

On the other hand, there would certainly have been far fewer mental health issues in an ancestral environment, as is still the case in modern-day hunter-gatherer cultures. People who live close to the earth have far fewer worries, far less work and far more rest, as well as a species-appropriate diet plus more restorative sleep.

It is therefore likely that most of us would have been in top condition most of the time. Our Paleolithic period did represent the peak of humanity, at least at its healthiest and happiest.

If the story of Paleo life seems romanticized to you, ask why. Why should the idea of being free and interdependent, unbound by arbitrary rules, having all you ever need while living in harmony with nature cause such a reaction?

Yes, it does sound idyllic, but that does not mean it is unrealistic. Surely the reason *why* we have such a deep emotional response is precisely *because* that way of living is embedded in our genes.

Humanity thrived harmoniously in the Paleolithic era for around 200,000 years. Working on a typical procreation timespan of twenty years per generation, it works out that, if you have had ten thousand ancestors, nine thousand five hundred of them lived that way. It is only the most recent five hundred at most who knew anything else. You are still fundamentally a stone age human but you are living in a world that looks very different.

In addition to getting a feeling for stone age life, there are a few very important points to take away from this chapter, which will provide the backdrop to everything that has happened since.

Understand that in nature, resources go to where they are needed, after which they are recycled again and again.

The cycles follow a natural pattern of in and out, similar to your breathing.

Fat cells absorb energy and toxins after a feast and then release them during the subsequent fast.

In a similar way, the tribe gathers more resources in the warm months that are then released again during the wintertime.

There are natural limits that prevent too much gathering of resources, thereby checking excessive growth. Any population is limited by the constantly changing availability of resources, whether land or vegetation or prey. If a group grows too populous, it risks over-harvesting, which could lead to scarcity, which would in turn cause a reduction in population.

That tendency to balance is nature's way, and we can see it has led to incredible variety, diversity, and richness. But note that, following nature's laws, the abundance is shared by all life.

However the natural balance, which had held all living things in constant harmony since the emergence of life on Earth, was about to be shattered, triggered by a sudden change in the climate.

Chapter 5:
A New Climate

It is believed that, somewhere around two million years ago, our early human ancestors migrated out of Africa and proceeded to colonize most of the land on Earth, eventually reaching every continent except Antarctica. This meant adapting the way they lived to different environments and to the seasons, which became harsher the further from the equator they traveled.

The last hundred thousand years of the Paleolithic era saw an ice age that left much of the land blanketed with glaciers and the resulting drop in sea levels created a land bridge that allowed humans to cross the Bering Strait into the Americas.

Our big brains, tools, weapons, fire, and language had made us into formidable hunters. However our hunting success was always constrained by the natural limits that help to hold populations of predators and prey in perpetual balance.

That state of harmony endured until around twenty thousand years ago and the start of the Neolithic Age (which means "new stone age"), when the last ice age began to give way to the current warm interglacial period.

As a direct result, the majority of humans on the Earth were forced to undergo a radical and rapid transformation in their diet, and consequently in their entire way of life.

The ice age had supported a variety of enormous land animals, the *megafauna* that included mammoths, giant ground sloths, and wooly rhinos, but these huge beasts all disappeared from the face of the Earth around the same time.

There is ongoing debate about what killed off the megafauna. Some argue that it was down to human hunting. Perhaps the warming climate drove the giant ice age beasts into ever-diminishing enclaves, making them easier to trap.

Others point to theories that an environmental cataclysm, known as the Younger Dryas impact event, believed to have occurred in the region of Greenland or North America around that time, could also have contributed.

Maybe all those factors played their part, and ultimately it does not really matter. However we can be sure of the outcome: the world was now significantly warmer and there simply were not enough large animals left to continue to support the human population in our ancestral hunter-gatherer way of life, except in a few regions.

At this time it is thought that there were still only around five million humans spread over much of the Earth's fifty million square miles of land outside of Antarctica. Population density had always previously been limited by the availability of game to a maximum concentration of one individual per square mile, which is the same as we still see today in those hunter-gatherer populations that retain their stone-age lifestyles.

As the world warmed up the great forests retreated, giving way to expanses of grassland, which tend to favor smaller herbivores. Smaller, faster prey meant hunting became more challenging, which is why we tamed wolves and bred them into dogs that could help us to hunt. (In fact the English word "hunt" is simply the German for "dog".)

Aside from their speed and agility, smaller game presented Neolithic humans with another problem: *leanness*. Small animals tend to have far less body fat than larger ones. For example, the meat on a deer comprises seventy percent protein and only thirty percent fat. Because humans cannot extract energy efficiently from protein we can only use a maximum of ten to fifteen percent protein in our diet (because the process of breaking down protein as fuel uses 25-30% of the energy gained, compared to only 2-3% for fat). That means we could only realistically make use of *less than half* of a small prey animal, and the rest would go to the dogs.

That is when the balance tipped. There still were animals out there that could be hunted in the wild, but over time we came to find it easier to feed ourselves from new, alternative sources.

As our likely ancient ancestor, Australopithecus, had been an omnivore, humans have always retained the ability to get some energy and limited nourishment from plant sources, as well as from animals.

We adapted our diets once again, but this time over a dramatically shorter timescale. Within just a few millennia, most of the human race transitioned from a hunter-gatherer existence to one based on *agriculture*. And applying our big brains and creativity to this new food source would come with disastrous consequences!

The need for new food sources drove the invention of agriculture to occur at various times in different parts of the world. Current evidence points to its having emerged in Asia around fifteen thousand years ago; in the region of the Mediterranean more recently, around five thousand years ago; but remarkably it only reached England two thousand years ago and Scotland another five hundred years after that!

Agriculture was only made possible because we discovered the process of *domesticating* plants from natural, wild ancestors into varieties that are more suitable for use as human food. There is evidence of the domestication of many different types of plants occurring independently in many regions of the world, but even the very earliest clues only go back a maximum of fourteen thousand years.

The result is that, over a span of several millennia in the Neolithic age, the dietary fuel make-up of most of humanity was turned entirely on its head. We switched from getting most of our food from meat to the majority coming from plants and in doing so we also flipped our macronutrient profile, from getting the bulk of our dietary calories from fat throughout the Paleolithic to carbohydrates in the Neolithic.

That change in our macronutrient intake is actually crucial to the story of humanity's degeneration. It caused radical and far-reaching changes, not only to our own lifestyles, but also to our health, to the way that we relate to each other, and even to the world around us.

One new type of food source in particular was responsible for the most profound change in our way of eating, and represented the first major example of humankind's domination of nature: *domesticated grains*.

There is evidence that Paleolithic humans had long supplemented their diets with some foraged wild grass seeds, which contain a little fat and protein along with starch. The earliest examples of Paleolithic stone tools that seem to have been used *specifically* to process plant-based foods are not particularly old, dating back between eighty-five thousand years in Africa and just forty thousand years in Europe and Asia.

But our grain consumption increased rapidly as we progressively bred various types of wild grasses into new strains that yielded far larger seed heads packed with more starch. The earliest example is believed to have been Emmer wheat, which was developed in an area in the Near East called the Fertile Crescent eleven thousand years ago, triggering what is now known as the *Agricultural Revolution.*

Selective breeding over many centuries enabled Neolithic humans to achieve higher and higher yields of starch. You can easily see the difference if you compare the seeds of any wild grasses growing in your area with the fat, swollen heads of modern wheat, barley, oats, or giant corn cobs. These novel, man-made inventions have been altered almost beyond recognition.

The ready abundance of *energy* in the new starch-rich grains meant they quickly became the staple food in most regions. Rice, for example, was first developed in Africa and then spread to Asia, whereas in Europe wheat, barley and rye were more successful. Corn emerged in what is now Mexico and spread to become the dominant food source in the Americas.

The reason why grains took over as humanity's number one food source is simple: they can provide *far more calories from less land*, which means you can fuel more people. That explosion in energy supply could then support a massive leap in population density from the previous natural constraint of one individual per square mile to *ten per square mile,* or even more!

It is hard to overstate the significance of this change, because it is the foundation for every subsequent development in recent human history, as well as being the catalyst for our degeneration and demise.

Using grains as the basis of our food supply in turn gave rise to *settlement*. Instead of following the herds, now we had food that could be reliably obtained in one place. As our major food source no longer ran away or migrated, we no longer needed to keep moving either.

In place of being dependent on the *herds*, we then became tied to the *land*. Starting the process of farming requires a significant up-front investment of labor, initially to clear the land of trees and rocks followed by the constant ongoing work of tending, weeding, planting, and harvesting crops. Obviously, anyone who invests all that time and energy to create a field will believe they are entitled, quite literally, to reap the returns.

The result was a profound shift within the human psyche. For the first time in our history, that piece of land became "*my* field".

As a result, we changed from knowing that we belonged *on the land* to believing that *the land belonged to us*. Suddenly the concept of *property* was no longer restricted to the small items, tools, and shelters that we made with our own hands, but now applied to the very earth beneath our feet.

In 1755 the philosopher Jean Jacques Rousseau came to that very conclusion in his seminal essay on the origins of human civilization, titled *"Discourse on the Origin and Basis of Inequality Among Men"*.

"...it is impossible to conceive how property can come from anything but manual labor: for what else can a man add to things which he does not originally create, so as to make them his own property? It is the husbandman's labor alone that, giving him a title to the produce of the ground he has tilled, gives him a claim also to the land itself, at least till harvest, and so, from year to year, a constant possession which is easily transformed into property."

Rousseau went on to identify the concept of land ownership as the defining factor that inevitably led to the demise of the human condition.

"The first man who, having enclosed a piece of ground, bethought himself of saying 'This is mine,' and found people simple enough to believe him, was the real founder of civil society. From how many crimes, wars and murders, from how many horrors and misfortunes might not any one have saved mankind, by pulling up the stakes, or filling up the ditch, and crying to his fellows, 'Beware of listening to this impostor; you are undone if you once forget that the fruits of the earth belong to us all, and the earth itself to nobody.'

...The poets tell us it was gold and silver, but, for the philosophers, it was iron and corn, which first civilized men, and ruined humanity."

There is clearly some truth in Rousseau's damning argument, not least in the fact that it soon led to the first evidence of *degeneration* in the human physical condition.

When anthropologists compare the skeletal remains of Paleolithic and modern humans, they consistently note a marked decrease in both height and body size of around ten percent.

As Marta Lahr, the co-director of Cambridge University's Leverhulme Centre for Human Evolutionary Studies, describes:

"When modern humans, Homo sapiens, first appeared around 200,000 years ago they were tall and muscular. The fossil evidence for the next 190,000 years is patchy, but shows that humans remained tall and robust until about 10,000 years ago when many populations show reduced stature and brain size. It is a striking change."

In more recent times, following the massacre of North American bison by the Europeans, the sudden impact was measurable on the Native American populations who depended on the bison. When physical anthropologist Franz Boas collected data on over fifteen thousand Native Americans between the years 1889 and 1919, the mean height was reduced by an average of over one inch. In addition, children who had been born after the bison slaughter grew up to be almost two inches shorter at adulthood.

The cause of this physical devolution should now be obvious. While we were generally getting plenty of energy to keep us alive, the food we were consuming was lacking in nutrients and so could not deliver the full complement of building blocks required to grow and maintain a perfect human form. The lack of essential fatty acids in the plant-heavy diet easily explains the sudden ten percent drop in brain size that accompanied the Agricultural Revolution.

Fossil records reveal that this degeneration affected more than just our physiology. This is also the period when we start to see the first evidence of nutritional deficiencies and chronic disease. The differences are so clear that an anthropologist can immediately tell whether they are looking at hunter-gatherer or agricultural human remains.

Paleopathology is the study of evidence of disease in ancient civilizations from preserved remains. The Ancient Egyptians left a particularly generous amount of evidence of health in the Neolithic era due to the number of mummies they preserved.

The Ancient Egyptian civilization, which emerged around five thousand years ago, lived on a diet primarily consisting of bread made from cultivated wheat, as we can see from the many wall paintings and sculptures that remain. We also know they consumed a variety of oils, which they pressed from a range of plant sources including olives, safflower, sesame, and flaxseed.

Analysis of mummified remains reveals the earliest known evidence of atherosclerosis and heart disease, in addition to polio, kidney disease, arthritis, tuberculosis, gout, tooth decay and more. We also know from their writings that the Egyptians recognized the symptoms of heart attacks.

What's more, the stone statues of wealthy persons show that rich Ancient Egyptian men tended to be fat and round and often even displayed evidence of gynecomastia (aka "man boobs").

One remarkable paleopathology study carried out in the 1970s proved to be exceptionally revealing, because it was able to analyze *side-by-side* large numbers of skeletal remains from two groups that had lived in the same area of western Kentucky. The two groups were likely to have been genetically identical and to have experienced very similar environmental conditions.

The key difference is that one was a non-nomadic hunter-gatherer tribe that had lived around five thousand years ago, whereas the other was an agricultural community that had farmed in the area during the sixteenth and seventeenth centuries, prior to contact with European settlers.

When comparing nearly three hundred skeletons from each of the two groups, the researchers discovered far more evidence of a range of health issues in the agricultural community.

While both groups seemed to have experienced periodic times of malnutrition, the remains of the farmers showed they suffered *far more* from anemia, infections, arthritis, tooth decay and tooth loss, as well as having lower life expectancy and higher infant mortality.

Another unpleasant side effect of our new way of feeding ourselves was that we now had to do *a lot more work*. The days of being able to support ourselves in full health with only a couple hours of exertion each day had come to an abrupt end.

Looking on the bright side, we had managed to create a fairly reliable supply of food, which would be able to sustain the growing human population indefinitely in the new warmer climate.

In the simplest terms, humanity made the change from living and sourcing our food *extensively*, when we roamed and hunted over a large area of land, to living and sourcing our food *intensively*, extracting far more from less land.

Except there was a problem. Agriculture could *not* sustain us indefinitely, due to a fundamental flaw in the system: a flaw so critical that it would cause the collapse of multiple empires, yet so slow to manifest that we would not figure it out for several thousand years.

Chapter 6:
Killing the Earth

We are constantly being told that "killing the planet" is a modern problem that only started to manifest after the industrial age, but that is not the case. In fact humanity started to destroy the Earth's biological diversity and fertility when we first tilled the soil.

When the climate warmed up and we moved from being mainly nomadic hunters to settled farmers, the resulting shift from getting most of our energy from carbs from plants in place of fat fundamentally changed the way we related to the land.

And the reason relates to the relative properties of those two forms of macronutrient. From any given area of land, carb-rich plants like grains and potatoes deliver *far more energy* than you can get from animal fat.

Of course, back when we traded big guts for big brains, we gave up the means of extracting or synthesizing all the nutrition we needed from plants. We only retained the ability to get energy from the carbs they contain, along with some vitamins and minerals. We could no longer synthesize the essential fatty acids.

That is *the single direct cause* of the nutrient-deficiency and resulting rapid degeneration of the human race over the past ten thousand years, which goes far beyond just our physiology.

As a species, we got addicted to this new intensive way of life, with our novel fuel source and the rapid growth it could power… in fact that growth was inevitable.

It is a simple fact that we can get *massively* more energy from the land by growing crops, compared to raising livestock. For example, modern wheat can provide more than six million calories per acre each year, while a potato crop can yield almost three times that amount. In comparison, pastured beef delivers only in the region of 160,000 calories per acre annually, only around *one percent* of the energy you can get from potatoes.

Now, calorific value should never have been, and should never be, the sole unit of measure when thinking about food. We need nutrition as well as energy in order to live and to be healthy, and these carb-rich crops deliver far too much of one, but far too little of the other.

Fatty meat is the ideal human fuel, providing both all the energy and nutrients you need, but crucially it takes more land *and* more time to build that fat. Prior to the agricultural revolution, humans had accessed fuel from both animal and plant sources according to what nature provided through the year, relying on extensively-sourced animal products for most of the solar cycle, but gorging on the extra fat-promoting calories provided by plant sources in the build-up to winter.

Consider that a hunter-gatherer would not have had constant access to carbs in nature. There are short periods each year when bushes may be heavy with berries and some trees might bear fruit. At other times, you might dig up a particular tuber, like the Hadza of Tanzania do today. Or perhaps you would be lucky enough to come across a bees' nest which you could raid for its sweet honey.

While these foods might be very welcome, giving a short-term energy boost, although admittedly little nutritional value, they could never have provided our everyday sustenance. We were still compelled to get most of our food by hunting, which meant our food supply was constrained by the natural limits of the availability of prey and the importance of maintaining balance, hence limiting our population density to one square mile each.

But what about tribes like the Tukisenta people of Papua New Guinea? Don't they get the vast majority of their calories from yams? Yes, absolutely, but the Tukisenta are a *Neolithic* people who can only access enough calories that way by farming using Neolithic methods. Yams (or sweet potatoes) are modern cultivars of a type of wild vine, which seem to have been domesticated independently in the Americas, Africa, and Asia, but all during the Neolithic era. They were probably introduced to Papua New Guinea by Europeans only a few hundred years ago. And, of course, the Tukisenta still rely on seafood for their essential nutrition.

Crucially, the move to agriculture eradicated the natural limits to human population density. Instead of foraging for occasional tubers and grains, domestication meant we could plant *monocultures*: entire fields of the same thing. That's how we managed to squeeze *far more energy out of far less land*, which meant that the factors that had previously constrained population density and population growth were radically rewritten.

Now, instead of depending on the herds of slow-growing and mobile prey, our food source was fast-growing and static. The factors limiting how much food we could extract from our environment now shrank to just two: available land, and available labor.

As previously mentioned, agriculture is hard work. However when it is successful it provides a huge bounty of calories, therefore it made sense for humans to breed more frequently, with more hands making lighter work.

As the population grew, fuelled by the abundant carbohydrates, we could continually clear more land and plant more crops. There was nothing to hold us back, until we came up against rocky and mountainous terrain or a large body of water.

So over time, we continued to grow in numbers and in density as we turned most of the available land over to cultivation and developed more efficient farming techniques. No longer limited to one square mile per individual, the ever-expanding population started to concentrate in villages, then towns, eventually leading to city-states. Humanity had entered the age of *civilization*.

But every civilization that ever existed was built on the same type of fundamentally flawed accounting, which is why no empire has ever endured for more than a few thousand years.

There are many reasons why we have repeated the same pattern, but the core problem is that the destruction of civilization is invisible, and that's because it happens beneath our feet.

It turns out that we have been "killing the planet" for thousands of years, and we walked blindly into our own demise for one simple reason: *arable agriculture is unsustainable*.

In fact, the means of our destruction happens to be the very same tool that enabled our meteoric growth: *the plow*.

Early Neolithic Man discovered that turning the soil not only helped to manage weeds but also caused a boost in fertility, which meant crops grew better.

But that increase in fertility is in fact an illusion, because it actually happens as the result of destroying soil-dwelling organisms. Science has only relatively recently discovered that the soil beneath our feet is far from just a layer of inert minerals, but a breathtakingly complex ecosystem of its own, which supports an incredible array of life.

Every time soil is tilled, it physically damages a vast number of living things, including animals like worms as well as complex subterranean fungal webs. Turning the soil exposes it to the air and sunlight, also killing incalculable numbers of tiny animals, bacteria, and other microbes.

All these dead organisms then release their stored nutrients, in particular *nitrogen*, which is crucial for plant growth, and that is what causes the apparent increase in short-term fertility, but it comes at the cost of long-term soil health. The problem is that the resulting soil degeneration manifests relatively slowly. It takes hundreds of years, but with continual tillage the earth eventually loses its ability to support life. The soil eventually turns into dirt.

Consider that you rarely see bare soil in a healthy, abundant natural environment. By definition, wherever there is exposed soil, nothing is growing. Where natural life is flourishing, the soil will also be concealed, covered by a "skin" of decaying organic matter. That layer protects the soil from the elements and provides shelter and food for a myriad of life forms. Why would it make sense to ignore the perfect model that nature has created for us and decide that it must be preferable to upturn the soil and expose it to the air?

Bare soil is, by definition, a sign of the desertification process. When the earth is overturned and compacted by the plow, it also loses some ability to absorb the vital rainfall, leading to runoff that washes soil downhill, where it eventually ends up in rivers and oceans.

When you study how and why agriculture works in terms of nature's models, it is easy to see why it is so destructive. To put it into context, we need to understand the natural cycle of *succession*.

Any land will, at some point, have to start from barren dirt, as it takes a long time to build soil. So the starting point is relatively inert: sand, clay, or silt that contains hardly any life-giving organic matter.

Nature's first step is to send in pioneer plants, otherwise known as annuals. These are the plant kingdom's opportunists and they propagate by spreading large numbers of seeds, which can lie dormant until some event triggers them to try to start growing, initially using their stored energy.

Annual plants serve an important role in bridging the gap between desert and self-sustaining fertility. Because they are small plants and only have shallow roots, they are able to cling on in the most inhospitable environments. Think of the weeds growing in cracks in the concrete, for example. But at least their meager roots help to start to bind the dead dirt together and give it a little more ability to store moisture. When they die after one season, they add a small amount of organic matter to the early-stage soil.

In that way, the pioneering annuals help to create the conditions for other plants, the longer-lived perennials. These are larger plants, the shrubs, bushes, and trees that have a longer-lasting influence on the environment. Because perennial plants need to survive for more than one year, they need more nutrients and water, and that means they need to push longer roots deeper into richer soil.

Of course some soils are not rich or moist enough to support many bushes or trees. These areas will be colonized first by annuals, including annual grasses, which will then be overtaken by perennial grasses. Note that perennial grasses, which naturally occupy the vast majority of the world's various grasslands, are quite different from their short-lived annual cousins, able to put their roots several feet down into the soil, rather than just a few inches in the case of annual grasses.

Over time, as soils grow deeper and richer, other larger perennials may take over, the huge trees that create forests and jungles. They may persist until some cataclysmic event, such as a fire, flood, earthquake, or mudslide destroys the ecosystem and resets it to bare dirt, when the cycle of succession starts over once again.

You may be wondering how all this affects agriculture. The answer is that all our staple row crops, from potatoes to corn to wheat, are *annual plants*. They are fast-growing but short-lived. Their shallow roots help them grab some available resources in a limited time, which they store in their reproductive parts: tubers (in the case of potatoes and other root vegetables), or seeds (in the case of legumes and grains). Those energy-rich "children" of the annual plants are what humans learned to harvest for their higher concentration of calories.

But, once you understand the cycle of succession, you can spot a fundamental problem. Annual plants cannot hope to compete in established, rich ecosystems, against established plants with deeper roots. They are niche opportunists and they actually need desert-like conditions.

And that is what the plow provides. Tilling the soil removes other plants that may compete with the desired row crop, together with a plethora of other life forms and releasing a burst of apparent fertility in the process. Once the crop has grown, stored its energy, and been harvested, it is time to repeat the process. Back comes the plow, and the soil is once again reset to square one.

In this way, the practice of agriculture is really no more than executing an artificial environmental catastrophe every few months, like continually hammering a big, red button marked "RESET". Any efforts that life might make to try to get established must be repeatedly wiped out, over and over and over again. In this way, agriculture simply and inevitably *kills soil*.

Of course, our Neolithic forebears did not know any of this, as it took centuries to kill off the lush soils they inherited from previous ages. So they continued to till. They went from hand tools to plows pulled by humans and then figured out how to harness the power of domesticated animals such as oxen and horses to work more land in less time.

Because intensively-farmed grains provided more energy from the land, it also made economic sense to feed our draft animals on grains and by-products that were inedible by humans. As well as requiring less land for extensive grazing, farmers also discovered that a diet high in grains would make animals fatter and therefore tastier when they came to slaughter.

With every pass of the plow, the soil's fecundity *appeared* to increase, but it came at a price as its long-term vitality took a hit.

Nature obviously builds soil, but it occurs at a very slow rate. It takes on average around five hundred years to create just a *single inch* of topsoil. Other factors mean that soil is also naturally eroded, but the worldwide average rate of soil erosion, before human beings started farming, was estimated to be one inch every one thousand four hundred years, which would therefore result in a net gain.

However pre-industrial agriculture tilted the balance dramatically. The invention of the plow sped up the rate of soil loss to *one inch every sixty years*, around ten times quicker than the soil can naturally generate!

If we take the typical depth of topsoil, which tends to be between eight and sixteen inches, we can calculate that, once humans started to till the land, it would only take between five hundred to one thousand years to deplete completely the soil in any particular area.

Think of plowing the soil as being like making withdrawals from a long-term savings account that offers a low interest rate. Without being able to see the balance you will not notice any change, but eventually the account will inevitably run out of funds.

Another important factor here is the human lifespan. In any population, the combined *living memory* of all generations currently alive might reach back around a hundred years. If it takes five hundred or more years for the soil to lose its fertility, we simply would not notice.

One of the meanings of the word "cultivate" is to tend or nurture. But agriculture does not nurture the earth, in fact it is closer to *soil mining.*

Without knowing it, our immediate gains would come at the expense of the population's long-term interests, leading to inevitable ruin. The soil would eventually become lifeless and therefore could no longer support a human population.

We've had this evidence right in front of us for millennia. Ultimately we would figure out what we were doing, but not until the modern day, and in the intervening time many empires would have to suffer a similar fate.

Historians have long speculated on what caused every previous empire on Earth to fall into oblivion.

It was an outlier named David R. Montgomery, a professor of the science of geomorphology who happened to become obsessed with soil, who finally pieced together the clues and realized that it was all down to soil mining.

When we look back at human history (the Holocene period, which spans from the end of the ice age to the present day), every great empire seems to have had a similar general lifespan: typically burning out in between 500 and 1000 years. Montgomery's contention, which he set out in his book *Dirt: The Erosion of Civilizations*, was that each one has risen and then expired as it destroyed its topsoil.

The Roman Empire, for example, conquered dozens of other nations and used the newly occupied land to grow food, yet it endured for only 507 years.

We also know that the Romans used to source much of their food from North Africa, including olives and cereal crops. The writer Tertullian, who came from Carthage, in what is now Tunisia, gave the following ominous account in 30 A.D.

"All places are now accessible, well known, open to commerce. Delightful farms have now blotted out every trace of the dreadful wastes; cultivated fields have overcome woods... We overcrowd the world. The elements can hardly support us. Our wants increase and our demands are keener, while Nature cannot bear us."

You may be surprised to learn that, at that time, northern Africa was dubbed, "the granary of the world". Now that region has another name: the Sahara desert.

When soil becomes dirt and loses its ability to support plant life, the rapid cycle of desertification kicks in. Plant cover creates a cooling effect in the atmosphere, which encourages precipitation. If there is no vegetation there will be very little rain, and if it doesn't rain no vegetation can grow.

"It was in an American desert that I suddenly realized that rain does not fall from the heavens – it comes up from the ground. Desert formation is not due to the absence of rain, but the rain ceases to fall because the vegetation has disappeared." ~ Masanobu Fukuoka, The One Straw Revolution

Consider also the area of the eastern Mediterranean previously known as the Fertile Crescent. Dubbed "the cradle of civilization" it is where the Neolithic Agricultural Revolution is thought to have started, in turn giving rise to many great empires.

The Fertile Crescent spanned modern-day Syria, Lebanon, Jordan, Palestine, Israel, Egypt, and parts of Iraq, all of which, again, are now mostly arid.

We find the same story over and over again: with the Mesopotamians, the Minoans, the Mayans, the Incas, as well as the Ancient Greeks. Plato wrote in the fifth century B.C.E., "The rich, soft soil has all run away leaving the land nothing but skin and bone."

Every one of those once great civilizations expired within a similar timeframe.

One notable exception was the Ancient Egyptians, where the Pharaohs ruled for a record three thousand years. The difference was due to a particular geographic effect in which every year the river Nile would flood, as rains washed fresh topsoil down from the Ethiopian plateau, which continually restored the delta's fertility.

Montgomery shows how all the great empires were forced to expand due to predictable soil depletion, eventually reaching some limit, such as an ocean or mountain range, or another competing empire. Like fire burning through a sheet of paper would reach the edge, each one would eventually burn out and disappear into the history books, leaving the earth to start the slow process of regenerating.

For millions of years, our ancestors had lived in a state of harmony with their natural environment. With the advent of the plow, we were now locked into a pattern of self-destruction that starts with obsessive expansionism but results in inevitable ruination every time.

Wherever you look in nature, you can observe awesome complexity and beauty. That complexity comes about through the action of sometimes competing, sometimes complementary forces that ebb and flow in cycles.

Nature's patterns are characterized by being in constant flow. Without flow, there would only be entropy and lifelessness, which is a state beyond death. Too much energetic flow, on the other hand, could lead to chaos that would also be unable to support life. The universal laws seem perfectly designed to walk the line between entropy and chaos, maintaining everything in a beautiful state of balance, and allowing life to go on.

We are all constantly subject to a host of natural cycles, including breathing in and out, night and day, the changing of the seasons, weather patterns, life and death, and the movements of the sun and the moon, just to name a few.

We have also touched on several more already in this book, such as the swelling and contraction of population numbers, how the availability of food led to feasting and fasting, and the resultant in-and-out action of our fat cells.

It seems now that the romantic view of pastoral life may hide a darker problem. We believe that our current way of life as a species has a future, but does it? Is there any way to avoid suffering the same fate as all previous agriculture-based human civilizations?

The first step to recovery is to admit that you have a problem. If we are to have any hope of a long future on Earth, we need to start by calling our current way of life what it really is: *unsustainable*.

It is obvious that any culture that cannot manage its resources in a sustainable way also cannot hope to survive in the long term. Our present way of feeding our population clearly takes far more than it puts back, and that is not nature's way.

However, that is not quite true. There are *some* organisms known to science that take resources without giving back: parasites. Whereas most living things follow the natural, sustainable, cyclical model, parasites simply keep taking and some can even kill their host.

Human civilization since the Agricultural Revolution has unconsciously been behaving very much like a parasite, constantly taking life from the earth without consideration for the health of our host. As a result our population growth has accelerated beyond control, and in recent times even went exponential. We are now at the point where we find ourselves faced with the prospect of having to feed ten billion mouths by the end of the current century. Yet our model for feeding ourselves is clearly doomed to failure.

Our own modern day civilization seems locked into the same doomed pattern as the ones that rose and fell in years gone by, due to our ongoing addiction to agriculture and the cheap, abundant calories it supplies.

Modern humanity continues to behave like a parasite on the Earth, but almost nothing is being done to turn things around. We will go on to explore why, instead of halting or reversing the System's parasitical growth, we are all playing our part in encouraging it to continue to expand and consume more and more.

Humanity is not only rolling the dice once again, but we are doubling down on destruction! If it seems insane, it is! That we are not only continuing on a path that can only lead to ruin, but that we are accelerating toward it, is madness.

And that's because the inmates have taken over the asylum.

Chapter 7:
The Rise of the Psychopath

The switch to agriculture and the resulting invention of the idea of land ownership also led to a further sinister and insidious degeneration, which was in *the way we related to each other*.

Basing our diet on carbs not only gave rise to settlement and created far more work, but it also increased our *dependency on food*. From being able to go for days between meals, we became carb addicts who needed multiple daily fixes. (While we imagine that the idea of "our daily bread" must be ancient, it actually only entered into human consciousness within the last ten thousand years, that's just *five hundred generations*!)

A combination of the new phenomenon of private ownership of land together with a growing population that is dependent on a regular food supply fundamentally shifted the balance of power in human society, ushering into existence a two-tier system of haves and have-nots, in other words *owners* and a dependent *slave class*.

It can be argued that, if an individual is no longer able to survive without constant meals, and if they are also dependent on whoever owns the land that grows the food, they can no longer be considered *truly free*.

From this point in time, the attribute of owning arable (which means "plowable") land conferred onto the landowner a new degree of influence over the lives of others who did not own land. In place of our natural, ancestral state of interdependence within our tribe, suddenly some human beings found themselves dependent on others for their sustenance, their means of staying alive. Food was no longer out there for the taking; the *control of its supply* created an imbalance of power.

For the first time in our history, we encountered situations in which one individual had the right to *demand* labor from another.

To understand the impact of this rift that so divided the human race, it is helpful to introduce two models from *economics*: the study of the distribution of resources.

We have already seen how it is nature's way to tend towards cycles that maintain harmony and balance. For example, if predators multiply in number, they can then hunt more prey animals. That could mean the prey population in turn reduces, thereby making it harder for the predators to hunt, which again might result in a drop in the predator population, maintaining balance.

In economics and science, that pattern is what is called a *normal distribution*. In a normal distribution, the tendency is to pull towards the *center*. For example, the height, shoe size, and IQ of human beings are all distributed according to the familiar *normal* bell-shaped curve.

However there is an alternative, very different model for the distribution of resources, which does occur in a few select cases in nature, and which also happens to have become the dominant model in our modern human civilization.

In 1906 an Italian economist named Vilfredo Pareto noticed that, wherever he looked in society, eighty percent of wealth and property belonged to just twenty percent of the population. What's more, the effect was logarithmic, in that, among that top twenty percent, the top twenty percent of those individuals (i.e. 4% of the population) owned eighty percent of that wealth (64% of all the wealth), and so on.

The same pattern could also be observed in many other areas of life, and soon became known as the Pareto Principle, or the 80/20 rule.

You can observe the Pareto Principle in effect throughout modern society. The winner of the gold medal in an Olympic race might get far more fame and fortune than the runner who came in the silver medal position, even though the actual performance difference might be marginal. Most soccer players earn little or nothing, while a few thousand might be able to make a living at the game, and a small minority are super-rich. The same goes for artists, actors, writers, chefs, singers, and most other professions.

What Pareto had discovered was the opposite of the normal distribution, which we might call an *abnormal* pattern, in which, rather than to tend towards balance, resources in fact attracted more resources.

In a Pareto distribution, you could say that the pull is not towards the center, as it is in a normal distribution, but towards the *bottom*. In this model the majority have few resources and so find it difficult to fight the gravitational pull toward the bottom of the pile. However, those that do manage to succeed can go on to succeed to an extraordinary degree, because having relatively more of something actually makes it easier to get even more.

As it happens, the Pareto Principle does occur in nature, notably in the area of sexual reproduction and the phenomenon we call the survival of the fittest. For example, in many animal groups, mating rights go exclusively to the alpha male, who will vigorously defend his privileged position, ensuring that his genes are passed on more than his competitors'.

Pareto also tips the balance in favor of the strongest offspring. For example, a sow may give birth to more young than she has teats to feed them with, creating a situation of *scarce resources* and forcing the piglets to compete for food. If the weakest fail to get enough energy they often die. Likewise, parent birds will tend to give the louder and stronger of their chicks more food, again often leading to the death of the weakest.

While such aspects of nature may seem cruel to us, they are important for keeping populations strong and thus enhancing the overall richness and splendor of the natural world. It is also very likely that survival of the fittest played a part in our own ancestry. For example, in Greece in the Iron Age (much later than the Neolithic), we know the Spartans would sacrifice any babies that were born feeble or with physical deformities, so infanticide may well have been a feature of Paleolithic culture.

However, we must bear in mind that, even where Pareto does apply in nature, it nevertheless must always operate within the constraints of a greater, overriding normal distribution. Even though a pride of lions may get stronger over time, and even though they may outcompete other prides, they can never break out of the natural limits that prohibit overhunting (through the tendency to normalization of resources).

Paleolithic humans had always been bound to live within those same constraints. With regard to food, it wouldn't make sense to harvest any more than you would need, helping to ensure you get to the next time of abundance. If we chose to hunt more mammoths than we could consume, that would not mean we ultimately got *more* mammoth meat, but *less!*

Ancestrally, as long as the earth's fundamental fertility was maintained, you would only ever need enough to see you through.

Likewise there was no point in any individual crafting more arrowheads than the tribe could use, or that they could trade with other tribes. There was no point building a mud hut that was any bigger than was required to protect its occupants. Why spend all that time and energy for no extra benefit? Common sense dictates that our ancestors would invest their time and energy in sourcing or making only what they actually needed, so they could then focus on more enjoyable activities.

The key point is that, when we moved from hunting to farming, we broke away from most natural constraints. Suddenly, land ownership meant that Pareto's abnormal distribution took over from normal distribution as our default model for dividing resources, concentrating them into the hands of those who already have the most. As a consequence it also opened the door to another novel concept: *the class system*.

In Paleolithic times, if the strongest hunter decided to declare himself king and that, as king, he was going to keep all the mammoth meat to himself, within a few days it might have rotted, so there would be absolutely no benefit. (Apart from anything else, the rest of the hunters would probably have just kicked his royal butt!)

It therefore made much more sense for everyone to share, not just the hunters who made the kill, but the woman who fletched the arrows, the children who fetched the water and tended the fire, the healer who sourced the medicinal herbs, and the elders who entertained everyone at the feast with traditional songs and stories. In other words, sharing resources benefited the whole tribe, and when the tribe benefited, every member of the tribe benefited in turn.

In this way we had always lived by nature's *normal* balance. Everything we needed was there for the taking, and there was no advantage to anyone to take more than they needed.

What makes the difference between the normal and abnormal models is the *scarcity of a resource*. Whether the resource may be procreation rights, celebrity, or gold-medal-winner status, scarcity creates value.

In prehistoric tribal times, food was generally not a scarce commodity. It stands to reason that we were successful at finding food because we not only survived those times but thrived to spread right over the face of the Earth. Wherever humans settled, anytime they needed food, they just went out and hunted or gathered. Whatever they might require, whether wood, leaves, mud, sand, honey, herbs, moss, flint, bird feathers, or a shell, they would know where it was available in the local area and could simply go out and fetch it.

But after we settled into permanent agricultural communities, we could no longer just walk out into nature and get whatever we needed anymore.

And that is the start of The System, where the many become beholden to a few.

Ownership also created the possibility of unequal trades. Previously, if people from two different tribes wanted to trade some stuff for some other stuff, each party by definition must have placed a higher value on what they were getting than whatever they were giving up, otherwise the trade would not go ahead. That way everybody comes away a winner.

But now, for the first time in human history, a minority had power over the majority. If you had land and another did not, you could be in a position to demand they trade their labor in return for food. You could very likely force them to invest more effort than it would have taken their hunting and gathering ancestors to feed themselves.

Instead of getting returns based only on what you had *made or sourced* with your own time, which of course is subject to natural constraints, you could now be compensated simply for what you *owned*, which is not. That meant Pareto kicked in: those that *had* more could get more and more. The greater the number of individuals you could have clearing and working the land on your behalf, the faster you would profit, which meant you could potentially afford to acquire more land, and thus the abnormal distribution model amplifies.

This inequitable distribution of access to food surely also introduced a new form of emotional and psychological pressure.

In truly natural living, any lack or stress or injury would usually be short-term. You might hide from a threat, run away from it, or you might get eaten by it. Either way, the stress would be short-lived.

But now the new model of dependency created a new concept: poverty, and the possibility of living under sustained, chronic stress, something human populations had never previously endured.

For the first time, the new abnormal model where resources attract even more resources presented some individuals with the opportunity to hoard more than they could ever personally use. The new class of owners would also need to defend their "property", so they could hire guards to protect their stored wealth from anyone who might dare to attempt to help themselves to it.

You could say that the first grain to be stored in a barn was the first form of wealth. In due course, the Neolithic invention of money simply abstracted that wealth into a more portable form.

Previously, in ancestral times, the amount of anything that anyone could own was constrained by certain natural limits: their skill, the number of daylight hours, local availability of resources... and then how much you could physically carry or store or protect!

With the flip into the Pareto model, together with the invention of currency, one individual could now conceivably own far more resources than they could ever personally produce or even use in their lifetime! Money meant that the potential for wealth could break out of any natural, *normal* limits and was now bound only by *numbers*... which of course are infinite!

But, considering our evolutionary history, you might ask why anyone would wish to harvest more resources than they could ever need? Why would they be so driven to wield power over others? One possible answer is that the invention of wealth created the concept of *status*. To use a phrase that has persisted to the present day, possessing wealth meant you were "worth more".

Even today, the majority of us who carry within our genes the memory of our ancestral ways have little desire to exert control over our fellow humans.

But there is one type of personality that lacks the normal, instinctive tendency towards free and equitable interdependence. From time to time an individual is born with a combination of three mental abnormalities. These are the personality disorders that make up what is known as *the dark triad*.

The first disorder is a lack of empathy, the inability to contemplate the impact of any course of action on the feelings of others. In the modern day, this might be called anti-social behavior disorder, sociopathy, or subclinical psychopathy.

The second disorder is narcissism. Narcissists have an overinflated sense of self-importance; they genuinely believe they are better, and deserve more, than other people.

The third is to have a lack of the scruples that normally prevent individuals from manipulating others for personal gain, which may involve charming, lying, or cheating.

When all three disorders are present, you have what we will refer to throughout this book as a *psychopath*.

In prehistoric life, trusting your tribe was not even an issue. Of course you would trust your fellow tribe members, not least because nobody had any reason to misrepresent the truth, to lie, cheat, or swindle anyone else. Because everyone generally knew what most others were doing, there would be nothing to police, and when all you might need was right there for the taking or making anyway there was no reason to steal.

But now, free from the natural constraints on population density, communities ballooned far beyond the tribal limit of around a hundred friendly faces. As a result, we lost the ability really to *know* everyone else. Now finding ourselves living side by side with strangers, the intrinsic tribal trust for everyone around you was no longer appropriate.

Add into the mix the opportunity for some individuals to gain power over others through the acquisition of wealth, we had unwittingly created the ideal environment for the psychopath.

As previously mentioned, in addition to lacking empathy, psychopaths tend to be *narcissistic*: believing they are more important than everyone else. They do not recognize their interdependence as part of a healthy whole and become more concerned with their own importance. So a psychopath would be particularly drawn to the pursuit of wealth and power, and the illusion of superiority they confer.

The other trait common in psychopaths is the willingness to manipulate others. Lacking normal moral restraint, they would be prepared to go to greater lengths to protect the perceived status that wealth brings, even at the cost of others in their community.

Arguably it is not wealth itself that is the problem, but rather what some people are willing to do in order to get it and protect it. As future scriptures would explain, "For the love of money is the root of all kinds of evil."

Now unshackled from tribal interdependence, lying, cheating, stealing, and swindling could be *profitable*.

In a healthy tribe, which lived by nature's laws that tend towards balance and harmony, any aberrant individuals who were unfortunate enough to be born with that particular set of deficiencies would have been removed. That would have been a necessity in order to maintain the overall integrity and health of the collective.

But in the new, larger, intensive communities, anonymity meant it was no longer easy to identify the faulty individuals. As a result, they were able to thrive, grabbing ever more wealth, power, and influence.

Soon, the psychopathic mentality would come to dominate the human species' entire way of life. It led us into an ever-accelerating, senseless competition to extract and hoard ever more resources.

Our move from extensive to intensive living had ignited a chain reaction of continual further intensification as the human population would concentrate in ever-greater numbers, and we would develop new ways to mine the earth even more efficiently. All the while, wealth and power would also continue to become further concentrated into fewer hands.

Within just a few millennia, that insane race for more, more, more would eventually lead to humanity facing a battle for its very survival.

We must realize that, for a few millennia, we have been behaving like a parasite upon the Earth, and we are also in danger of destroying the host.

But if most of us are not psychopaths, how did we come to organize our lives around a psychopathic model? The answer is that our very perception of reality, our sense of self, and our understanding of our place in the world have all been corrupted.

We now live in a society where our understanding of what is true and real has been replaced with a mutation: we now live in a world dominated by *bullshit*.

Chapter 8:
The Invention of Bullshit

In order to get the majority of human beings to accept living in a new model of society that encouraged greed and supported a two-tier class system, we would have to break away from the ancient, ancestral lore that reminded us of our intimate place within nature's cycles.

That break would trigger a cascade of radical changes in society that allowed its most ambitious and ruthless members not only to gain control over the food supply and most other resources, but also over the entire population, effectively reducing the majority of the human race into slavery. How the minority managed to achieve our enslavement is the greatest scam ever pulled off.

In this chapter we will describe that process, which involves a series of steps to strip away our sovereign freedoms and leave us dependent on The System.

The first step in our slide from freedom into slavery was to break our relationship to *truth*. For the first time in our existence on Earth, we would have to learn to accept what was not evidently real.

Tribal lore was our shared ancestral memory of how to do anything and everything for yourself, and hence for the benefit of the group, in harmony with the movement of the sun and the passing of the seasons. The lore had always been concerned with everything that was *real*.

While we have no way of knowing for certain, it makes sense that sun worship would likely have been the universal religion in the Paleolithic age, for the simple and obvious fact that the sun was and is evidently the origin and provider of all life. The sun's annual return in midwinter made the plants grow and thereby sustained all living things.

Our entire ancestral worldview was rooted firmly in reality: what we could see, touch, and experience directly for ourselves. For most of our existence, even the object of our worship had been visibly evident.

We had always *belonged to* the land, but the agricultural way of life depended on everyone agreeing to a new fiction: that the land *belonged to us*. For the intensive, agricultural Neolithic society, the old legends that had forever been our source of knowledge of where we came from and where we belonged now presented a problem.

While tribal wisdom spans past, present, and future, the psychopathic mind is concerned only with self-enrichment in the now. So the new model of society, built on unrestrained mining of the soil and the concentration of wealth that suited the desires of the psychopath, would have to be forced to celebrate short-term personal gain as a worthy objective.

That meant tribal lore would need to be uprooted and supplanted with *new rules* to govern how we lived.

Rousseau gave this account of the origin of law in his 1755 Discourse on Inequality:

"The cultivation of the earth necessarily brought about its distribution; and property, once recognised, gave rise to the first rules of justice; for, to secure each man his own, it had to be possible for each to have something...

"Such was, or may well have been, the origin of society and law, which bound new fetters on the poor, and gave new powers to the rich; which irretrievably destroyed natural liberty, eternally fixed the law of property and inequality, converted clever usurpation into unalterable right, and, for the advantage of a few ambitious individuals, subjected all mankind to perpetual labor, slavery and wretchedness."

The most fundamental reason for the invention of law was, and remains to this day, the need to protect property rights. While it is entirely understandable that we would have created rules that made it acceptable for individuals to lay claim to the land, that first law caused a drastic fracture in human mentality.

For the first time, accepting those original laws meant we must accept something abstract, something we could not *see* and verify with our own eyes, as true.

We had shifted into a new kind of existence where the real and the natural and the knowable existed alongside new, man-made laws that were abstract and arbitrary.

The invention of writing meant that, in place of oral tradition, which can evolve over time, our history, our religion, as well as newly-created laws could all be preserved in hard copy. The written word gave our rules permanence and credibility.

"Why aren't women allowed to go to stonings, Mum?" "It's *written*, that's why!" ~ Monty Python, Life of Brian

Philosophers have used many colorful terms to describe the overlaying of alternative, abstract realities on top of the real world that helps us to make sense of the senseless and keep the wheels of industry turning. It has been called fiction, false reality, pseudo-reality, or The Matrix, but the comedian-philosopher George Carlin's description is perhaps the most elegant: *bullshit*.

Carlin said that bullshit was "the American soundtrack" and described in his trademark style the essential role of false reality in maintaining societal cohesion:

"There's just enough bullshit to hold things together in this country. Bullshit is the glue that binds us as a nation. Where would we be without our safe, familiar, American bullshit?"

There always has to be just enough bullshit; the greater the difference in distribution of wealth, the more bullshit would be needed to justify it. The two go hand in hand.

In his book "On Bullshit", which is dedicated to understanding the distinctive features of that phenomenon, writer Harry G. Frankfurt takes as his starting point a previous essay by Max Black that describes the term "humbug" thus:

"HUMBUG: deceptive misrepresentation, short of lying, especially by pretentious word or deed, of somebody's own thoughts, feelings, or attitudes."

This offers some important insights into bullshit. Bullshit does not mean total falsehood. The key feature is its intention to misrepresent the *true intent* of whoever is in charge of delivering the narrative. Most political dialog, for example, is not made up of lies, much of it *seems to be* in the interests of the people. However, it belies the ultimate true intentions of The System of which it is a product, which is the constant appropriation of wealth by stealth.

Now that people are ready to accept the unreal as real, the second step in the creation of a slave class is to persuade them to allow *others* to set the rules.

Our history had always come from *us* and lived in our memory through oral tradition. Up to this point, the only sources of authority in tribal life had been the sovereign individual, the campfire council, tribal traditions, and ultimately the laws of nature that governed the whole living world.

The very act of accepting a deed that tells you someone owns a piece of land means you must agree there is another external authority that, aside from natural common decency, can rightfully prohibit you from abusing the landowner's rights.

But if *others* could now set the rules by which you must abide, who would those others be?

In ancestral times, our small tribes would have come to their own decisions in public. But with much larger, intensive communities, campfire councils were no longer feasible, so we had to introduce a further layer of abstraction in the form of representative decision-making. From that point on, important judgements would be made by a select few.

Whether we had much choice in the matter, handing over the making of laws to others was a further leap of faith, from which there would be no return.

We were now in a situation where we no longer had the authority to decide what was real anymore. That authority had become externalized. So whoever held control over those external sources now controlled our shared definition of reality.

The first judges were the wealthy landowners themselves, each ruling over his own territory. In various traditions the role of lawgiver was held by the chieftain or laird or yarl... invariably the richest and most powerful land-owning men.

Later, we developed the idea of representative democracy. In place of a sole ruler, the people's interests would be represented by others, the first politicians. True campfire democracy, which means "rule by the people", had been replaced with a bullshit facsimile: *democracy by proxy*.

Mutual trust has always been an intrinsic human trait, for the simple reason that, up to that point, it had always worked. Children would naturally trust what their parents or elders told them and would absorb a huge amount of practical knowledge in their formative years, which they would continue to refine in adulthood. Adults would in turn pass the lore on to younger generations, ensuring it was not lost and would continue to serve the tribe in years to come.

The introduction of bullshit left us in a state of permanent infancy with regard to our relationship to knowledge. We no longer had faith in ourselves, no confidence in our own discernment or in our direct experience of the real world. Instead, we would be kept stunted in a perpetual childlike state, dependent on authority to tell us what to think.

After eons of oral tradition, which passed knowledge down through the generations, we found ourselves locked into a world where a select few rulers, lawmakers, priests, and politicians have the authority and can therefore set the narrative. From that point, our definition of what was real and right would forever be dictated by others.

We had lost a fundamental liberty, but we couldn't be permitted to realize it. So the bullshit serves up an alternative reality that pretends we still have freedom. Even if life seems hard now, bullshit narratives implore us to labor on under the belief that there will be some end to our drudgery, perhaps through gaining enough wealth, or alternatively some reward in the next life.

What kind of individual would be drawn to wielding such power? The psychopath, who has the most to gain through acquiring wealth and status, and no conscience to hold them back.

"Society is like a stew. If you don't stir it up every once in a while then a layer of scum floats to the top." ~ Edward Abbey

A psychopath recognizes only his or her own needs and desires. In their world, they must do whatever serves and promotes their interests: wealth, power, status. No other course of action makes sense in a psychopath's mind. Other people simply don't matter, they are just things.

The truth is that laws do not ultimately represent the will and best interests of the People, but only the will and best interests of the *people who write the laws*.

Next, the Owners would need to find ways to sell the bullshit, make it easier to swallow.

When you are in a small minority it is surely not easy to maintain control over the majority. It is very difficult to ensure absolute domination through force alone. How could the Owners persuade the masses to consent to rules that clearly do not favor them, including removing their liberty and sovereign rights?

That's where the bullshit kicks up a gear. When the psychopaths took over they set about writing more rules that would mold human society into a System that in reality served the Owners' interests. Society could not be run for the benefit of all, yet it must be run to *appear to be* in the benefit of all.

In fact, selling bullshit to the common man did not prove to be too difficult of a challenge. Human beings have relatively short memories and we are naturally inclined to believe what we are told by authority figures (originally our parents and elders), as well as to recognize that we are responsible in some way for each other's well being.

Now separated from our tribal traditions and plunged into an anonymous world surrounded by strangers, we proved easy to fool. In fact, the art of bullshit even got its own manual!

The most complete, and most patently psychopathic, guide to dominating the masses was penned by the sixteenth century Italian politician Niccolò Machiavelli. The Encyclopaedia Britannica describes *The Prince* as...

"A short treatise on how to acquire power, create a state, and keep it, The Prince represents Machiavelli's effort to provide a guide for political action based on the lessons of history and his own experience as a foreign secretary in Florence. His belief that politics has its own rules so shocked his readers that the adjectival form of his surname, Machiavellian, came to be used as a synonym for political maneuvers marked by cunning, duplicity, or bad faith."

During his life Machiavelli only shared *The Prince* with select personal contacts, although it was published after his death. This quote is one example that illustrates his disdain for human nature.

"Any man who tries to be good all the time is bound to come to ruin among the great number who are not good. Hence a prince who wants to keep his authority must learn how not to be good, and use that knowledge, or refrain from using it, as necessity requires." ~ Machiavelli

One age-old solution to getting the people to swallow your bullshit is to put it in a sandwich, concealing falsehoods or untruths between slices of good sense and truth.

Psychopaths tend to be highly skilled in manipulation and have no problem with turning on the charm when there is something to gain (the trait psychologists call "Machieavellian"). They are also willing to perform good and generous deeds, which can be extreme and ostentatious, to reinforce the story that they must be good, but which in fact distract you from their other more self-serving activities.

In reality, a large part of the purpose of the political pantomime is to trick the people, by showing enough evidence of your good deeds, so that it becomes impossible for them to conceive that you could be capable of evil ones.

"Only six people in the Galaxy knew that the job of the Galactic President was not to wield power but to attract attention away from it." ~ Douglas Adams, The Hitchhiker's Guide to the Galaxy

The philosopher Hegel wrote that absolutely anything can be justified if we look hard enough for reasons. If you deliver your new rules in a package wrapped in solid reasoning and logic in a way that appears plausible, it only needs to *sound* good.

"The vulgar crowd always is taken by appearances, and the world consists chiefly of the vulgar." ~ Machiavelli

The package might include both negatives and positives. For example, "We must make these harsh cuts now in order to ensure future national economic security." Unappealing new laws might be mixed in with more attractive ones that offer the promise of some comfort, protection, or hope (which of course could either fail to materialize as promised or could be repealed later).

"The promise given was a necessity of the past: the word broken is a necessity of the present." ~ Machiavelli

You can also get buy-in by showing the common people how they actually benefit in some way from a new edict, but which in fact favors the wealthy elite to a far greater degree. Let's take the original fiction of land ownership. Thanks to the law protecting ownership, I get to say that this small piece of land is my land. But, if I fail to keep up payments on my taxes, my claim and property could be taken away from me. The same does not apply to the lord of the land.

Another reliable way to sell bullshit to the people is particularly insidious, and relies on a perversion of our natural instinct to interdependency, which had previously served us perfectly well. It is to appeal to "the greater good".

Collectivism is the concept that the group is more important than its individual members. The collectivism con works precisely *because* it is not total bullshit. It is based partly in truth, preying on our instinctive tribal memory of a time when we were interdependent, but that was when we knew and could rely on the faces around the campfire. In a larger society, interdependency breaks down.

Yet collectivism actually goes a step beyond natural interdependency, telling those of us who do care about others that the often intangible "greater good" is of *supreme* importance. Its great conceit is in telling us that, even in a large and anonymous society, we are *all* still responsible for *everyone*. That is how it has been used to trick us into serving the Owners under the false belief that we are helping each other.

Not only are we beholden to serve the needs of the abstract notion of "society", so our perception of society's needs can be manipulated by those who control information, but we are also all required to *believe* what (we are told) the majority believes.

As we have no way of really knowing what everyone in society wants, again we can only rely on authority, which implicitly represents the will of the community. So if we are told that something is generally accepted, we should also accept it unthinkingly. The more often something is repeated, the more it appears to be fact.

"The Party told you to reject the evidence of your eyes and ears. It was their final, most essential command... And if all others accepted the lie which the Party imposed—if all records told the same tale—then the lie passed into history and became truth." ~ George Orwell, Nineteen Eighty Four

Replacing true self-government with representative politics paved the way for that illusion of common agreement. Now that the political rulers were the arbiters of truth, the public could be fooled by the smokescreen of orthodoxy.

72

Ultimately, bullshit always benefits one particular type of individual most of all... the ones who get to make up the rules!

The System is set up to allow a few to benefit from the work of others. As we have seen, to ensure its continuation, the Owners must maintain the illusion that everyone is benefiting, even if that flies in the face of the evidence that the working classes are really slaves.

In order to prevent revolt, the new owners needed to back up their bullshit with *threats*, which would be both internal and external. The first of these was internal: society's laws needed to be *enforced*.

Under the collectivist illusion, injury against the State's laws constituted a threat to every one of its citizens, so it could not be permitted and should be publicly stamped out to ensure universal subservience. Non-compliance could not be an option. Everybody had to accept the external authority under threat of force: violence, or the loss of liberty.

Have we ever stepped back and asked why we really need law enforcement? Is its real purpose to protect and serve everyone? Or does it serve to maintain a specter of fear? In a free and just society, why would any one of us fear authority?

"It is much safer to be feared than loved because ... love is preserved by the link of obligation which, owing to the baseness of men, is broken at every opportunity for their advantage; but fear preserves you by a dread of punishment which never fails."
~ Machiavelli

Many thinkers, when contemplating the notion of violence, have commented on a strange phenomenon. Violence tends to be prohibited far more often when it is attempted by the weak against the powerful. Riots, rebellions, and direct action must always be swiftly quashed. However, when it is the powerful doing the damage, law enforcement is rarely the solution.

That's how countries can wage illegal wars without reproach, how corporations are free to destroy ecosystems in the name of progress or release medicines that result in mass deaths with impunity. Violence only seems to be a tool reserved for the powerful.

Is the reality that, despite the commonly accepted story that the law enforcers and military are there to protect the people's freedoms, they ultimately protect the rulers?

But what are they protecting themselves *from*?

It's us, me and you and our kids. The majority.

That's why society appears to be so divided in all kinds of ways. Left versus right, blue versus red, white collar versus blue collar, black versus white... But perhaps all these are bullshit false dichotomies whose real purpose is to distract us from the far more scary truth: that it's *them versus us*!

The real purpose of all the bullshit is to avoid revolt through maintaining control.

Those who do the actual work must always be in the majority. That is the key! They cannot control us through overt force alone, so they employ more sophisticated methods. Yet the threat of force must always be there in the background.

"Never attempt to win by force what can be won by deception." ~ Machiavelli

Is it unthinkable that we may not need this type of protection at all? People might protest, "If we had no laws and no police, society would collapse!" But whose society is it? If it is not really our society, but theirs, how great a loss would that be? Could we conceive of replacing it with a better alternative?

It was always true that our tribe was vital to the survival of its members, but that is not so anymore. Yet it serves the Owners for us to persist in a similar belief, so we had to be convinced of the vital need for protection. That's where *external threats* come in.

There is another grand false narrative whose sole purpose is to keep the people on edge. They must be constantly reminded that the world is a dangerous place!

Over the years society has been told it must fear foreign enemies, terrorism, immigrants, the threat of war, invisible pathogens, famine, the weather... the list goes on.

There is always a threat, but how real are they? How many have ever come to pass? Is it that the ever-present fear serves a vital purpose?

"You've got to be taught to hate and fear You've got to be taught from year to year It's got to be drummed in your dear little

74

ear You've got to be carefully taught." ~ South Pacific (Rodgers and Hammerstein)

Because they are convinced it is so perilous out there, the people not only accept but *demand* stronger leadership, more law and order, military, police, surveillance and espionage… all to protect us.

The Hegelian Dialectic, which can also be paraphrased as "Problem > Reaction > Solution", allows an abuser (or the State) to gain control by presenting a real or imaginary problem, from which the victim (or people) demand to be saved or protected, which is then promptly supplied. In fact, the solution often turns out to be a new problem!

Do any of those things actually make us more free, or is it just Stockholm Syndrome on a massive scale: the phenomenon where kidnap victims begin to feel sympathy and even love for their captors?

It is of course natural for parents to teach their children to respect authority, because parents are the authority in the family. In a tribal context, obeying your elders' instructions would have been an important survival skill that youngsters had to develop as soon as they could move independently.

But now, thanks to bullshit, our innate trust in our elders has been grossly expanded to apply to layer upon layer of faceless, external, unknowable authorities. No wonder one of the words we have for the System is "the nanny state", because, like a nanny, it plays the role of a substitute parent.

The assumption that we need leadership is yet another stretch into unreality born out of collectivism. The fact that we have society obviously means we need leaders… say our leaders. Representative democracy has been described as "the least worst system of governance so far discovered" but that is based on a massive presupposition. Do we actually need to be governed *at all*?

"I don't trust society to protect us, I have no intention of placing my fate in the hands of men whose only qualification is that they managed to con a block of people to vote for them." ~ Don Vito Corleone, The Godfather

In the guise of the protector who keeps us all safe, the psychopaths are in fact only seeking to protect themselves from *us*.

It is reasonable that at this point you might be experiencing a reaction to the idea that you are a slave. After all, you have freedoms! And that is true, but the big picture tells a different story. The freedoms we believe we have only operate within hard, set limits.

"None are more hopelessly enslaved than those who falsely believe they are free." ~ Goethe

If you are not free to walk upon the Earth and to live as you see fit, without harming others, you are *not free*, any more than a zoo animal that's "free" to move around its enclosure is free! If you ever have to question who is really the master of your life, *it isn't you*!

As we will see, as the System expanded to give the Owners ever more influence over the majority, the bullshit needed to get more and more all-encompassing, creeping ever closer to George Orwell's definition of totalitarianism:

"A society living by and for continuous warfare in which the ruling caste have ceased to have any real function but succeed in clinging to power through force and fraud."

Chapter 9:
Slave Food

We have seen how the dual inventions of agriculture and bullshit combined to create a System that split the human race into a two-tier power structure, built upon a culture of justified exploitation.

"But there's a reason. There's a reason. There's a reason for this, there's a reason education sucks, and it's the same reason that it will never, ever, ever be fixed. It's never gonna get any better. Don't look for it. Be happy with what you got. Because the owners of this country don't want that. I'm talking about the real owners now, the real owners, the big wealthy business interests that control things and make all the important decisions. Forget the politicians. The politicians are put there to give you the idea that you have freedom of choice. You don't. You have no choice. You have owners. *They own you!*" ~ George Carlin

Ever since the Neolithic era we have lived in a world where the flow of information is dominated by bullshit. All the world really *is* a stage. In fact, there are two coexisting realities: the theater that is presented to us, where we have freedom and opportunity; and the one behind the scenes, in which we are all ultimately serving a hidden cause, which is to give the Owners increasingly greater wealth and control.

The people labor on in the beliefs that society is set up in their best interests, that they are free, and that life is full of opportunity. This picture is at once *both true and false*. To the extent that it appears to hold true, that is only within limits.

When the chips are down, even though some individuals will prosper more than others, in the long term the house always wins.

It is only possible to maintain that grand illusion through the liberal application of bullshit. It is the classic carrot-and-stick scenario: we are encouraged to keep plodding forward by the carrot of being part of a stable, prosperous society that promises security and opportunity; we fear the stick of finding ourselves on the wrong side of our own laws.

Our rights, freedoms, and opportunities are only ours *on condition* that we behave and obey the rules. The penalties of violence or loss of liberty are always there in the background.

This should not come as a shock. Ever since the inventions of agriculture and wealth created the ideal breeding ground for the psychopath, society really could not have developed any other way.

The System *can* only ultimately serve the Owners, because it has at its core the Pareto Principle, which is fundamentally abnormal, so it has to replace nature's laws with a new reality modeled on the now-dominant parasitical and psychopathic persona.

The premise of this book is that the Owners have forever managed to keep the majority of people in a state of slavery by feeding them shit, which comes in two forms.

We previously explored the key role of bullshit in controlling our minds. But what of our bodies, and what part has food played in the perpetuation of mass servitude?

It is worth noting at this point that the System does not need to be judged, any more than we need to judge a psychopath. A psychopath works in the way a psychopath works. The System only needs to be *diagnosed* and it is plain to see that the System itself functions both parasitically and psychopathically.

As we know, a psychopath has an abnormally diminished capacity for empathy, an overactive sense of self-importance, and a readiness to manipulate others to serve their own needs. You can see that the System is set up to behave in the same way.

To the System, all resources are there for the taking, without regard to the impact on the wellbeing of other people, or the natural world. We have already seen that it has no scruples about falsehood; in fact lying has become an art form that spans many professions. In this psychopathic, self-serving System, compassion in others is simply a weakness, another resource that can be exploited.

It would be appealing to hope that society might weed out the psychopaths over time, however the opposite is true. That's because, due to the fact that wealth is so closely tied to status, it is in the interests of the psychopath to perpetuate their sickness through the generations.

Psychopathy is actually genetic and hereditary. You are either born a psychopath or you are not, and an individual that has psychopathy in their family history is more likely to exhibit psychopathic traits.

Psychopathic behavior can be mitigated, to some degree, if a child with these inherent tendencies is raised in a loving and nurturing environment. But that is less likely if the child is born, for example, into a high-status family that has always prided itself on a psychopathic way of life, that views itself as naturally superior, and identifies strongly with the wealth and status that it provides.

Furthermore, when status is tied to wealth, there will be the compulsion to preserve their wealth through the generations, because that reinforces the illusion of "natural" superiority.

If we accept that the System is by nature psychopathic, it must and can only serve itself, which means grabbing all the resources it can without consideration to the consequences.

As we have seen, the first vital resource was land that could be farmed to produce harvests, which equated to wealth.

While farming is far more productive per acre than hunting and gathering, it is also more labor-intensive. But of course the Owners cannot do all the work! Their role in the System is to profit continuously from the labor of *others*.

The whole System is built on a fundamental imbalance of power... in a very literal sense. Whereas previously, throughout most of human existence, the modest reward we took from nature was directly linked to the effort we expended, the new System is set up to deliver the greatest rewards to those who *do not do the work*.

The trick to making a surplus was to have *other people* working *your* land, each producing more output than they cost. That meant profits were constrained by a second scarce resource: *manpower*. The more intensively you wished to mine the fertility of the soil, the more manpower you would need. Even the use of power from draft animals, such as domesticated cattle and horses, still depended on human input.

But the problem with human beings is that they are slow to generate. A woman only usually makes one at a time, can only gestate once a year, and after that it takes many more years until the offspring reach an age when they can be useful to the Owner.

It is part of the psychopath's nature to view others as a subclass. If you are a psychopath faced with such a shortage of manpower, it makes much more sense to steal humans from somewhere else than to make your own.

One of the beautiful things for the Owners is that, compared to the rich hunter-gatherer lifestyle, the intensive agricultural approach required *significantly less skill*. For most tasks, simple, brute labor was all that was required. In fact, free thinking among your workforce was more likely to be a detriment.

"I don't want a nation of thinkers, I want a nation of workers" ~ John D. Rockefeller

While there is evidence that some humans dominated others and used them as slaves in ancestral times, its practice became commonplace following the move to agriculture.

"Mass slavery requires economic surpluses and a high population density to be viable. Due to these factors, the practice of slavery would have only proliferated after the invention of agriculture during the Neolithic Revolution, about 11,000 years ago." ~ Wikipedia

After all, in the psychopathic mindset, if something can be viewed as a mere object or possession, it is obviously just another resource to be exploited. So the Owners simply wrote new laws that stated who could be a slave, who could own slaves, and so on. Slaves became things because the law said so.

"He who has once begun to live by robbery will always find pretexts for seizing what belongs to others." ~ Machiavelli

Of course traveling to other parts of the world to capture slaves required a significant investment. That became more feasible—and profitable— as communities grew from villages into towns then into city-states, which could afford a full-time militia.

More labor meant more profit from the land. The desire to garner wealth from the available land will inevitably have led to competition between states. Those that could grow their resource base the fastest would be more likely to outcompete rivals, which created an incentive to mine the soil even more intensively.

The Bronze Age, and later the Iron Age, provided new technologies that benefited farmers as well as the military. Records of plowing soil go back as far as any written history. New metal blades made it possible to turn the soil more efficiently than ever, which of course only accelerated soil degradation.

We now know that this was the fatal flaw that halted the growth of, and eventually wiped out, every previous empire.

That of course would not matter to the psychopath. As long as there were new resources to be plundered, the soil mattered no more than people from other lands: they were all just things, and there was always more.

The problem, as we will continue to see unfold in the chapters that follow, is that, as the technological advances leaped forward, and our mining of the soil accelerated, our degeneration as a species also gathered pace.

But, if slavery was central to the parasitical growth of the System, where does food fit in?

Actually, food proved to be a highly effective tool for maintaining control over the slave class.

We have gone to lengths to stress the central role that food had always played in our natural day-to-day life. Food not only provided vital energy, but also nutrients and minerals to help keep our bodies strong, as well as building social cohesion.

It did not suit the Owners' objectives to have slaves who were alert, happy, and healthy. If their only value was in their basic physical output, they should be maintained in the lowest possible state of existence, and highest level of dependency, that still enabled them to carry out their chores.

That's why slave food was kept deliberately basic: cheap, quick, and empty of nutrients.

The first obvious benefit of course is purely economic. The psychopathic System does not care about the consequences to individuals as long as there are profits to be made. As slaves were no better than livestock, it only made sense to provide them with enough calories so that they could keep working, at the lowest possible cost.

Furthermore, it did not make sense for slave owners to give their slaves proper nutrition that might keep them in good health beyond their productive years. It not only did not matter if they survived into old age, but that could potentially constitute an unnecessary overhead.

A feeble slave is also more likely to be subservient. Feeding people a poor diet that lacks the proper nutrients their bodies need to build and to repair will impair both their physical and mental health, thereby keeping them weak. Dietary fats provide a kind of electrical insulation between brain cells, so a diet devoid of the right fats will lead to suboptimal brain function.

So what will they have been given? Simply the lowest-cost, mass-produced food that provided calories but little else. Just like with other livestock, slave diets have always been based on grains and other cheap crops.

Some have pointed to the fact that the gladiators in Ancient Roman circuses were referred to in texts as *hordearii*, which translates as "barley-eaters". They argue that, as the gladiators surely represented the elite athletes of their day, therefore a grain-heavy diet must have proven to be ideal.

There is some truth in that argument: the gladiators' diets probably were ideal... for their Owners! The majority of gladiators were slaves and so had very short life expectancy. Their diet of mainly barley and beans will have given them energy, and helped them to store fat as some protection against the horrors of the amphitheater, but long-term health simply was not as much of a factor as cost-efficiency.

It is much more telling to inquire what the rich—the landowners, politicians, and generals—ate, those who were in a position to choose for themselves. History provides plenty of detailed accounts of what wealthy Romans consumed at their feasts, and they point to an overwhelming preference for all kinds of meat, which often came from exotic sources.

A further aspect of our natural, self-sufficient lifestyle was that food was also a primary source of healing medicine. As the Greek philosopher Hippocrates said over 2000 years ago, "Let food be thy medicine, and let medicine be thy food."

The ability to source their own food meant that our ancestors could select from the larder that nature offered according to their bodies' needs from day to day. Like other animals, we naturally possess the ability to detect whether we might need more salt, more iodine, or more magnesium, for example, and would instinctively be drawn to foods that contained whatever was lacking.

Replacing self-sufficiency in a natural environment to a single, simple fuel supply also denied slaves the ability to self-medicate and thereby to maintain a balanced, healthful state.

Yet another reason to give slaves the most basic, ready-made gruel would be to curtail their emotional and social wellbeing.

Food is not only necessary for survival; it has always helped to build and maintain our visceral links to nature and to each other. Food is far more than a source of calories; it is a *process* that forms an important part of who we are at the most fundamental level. Our natural place in the world is to be self-sufficient, like every other living thing, free and able to go about sourcing what we need and want according to the season.

By definition, slaves are totally subject to their masters, which extends to removing their freedom to feed themselves. Being dependent on another for their food means a slave is no longer in that position of self-sufficiency: being able to select what they most need or desire. Denying entirely slaves' ability to source their own nourishment is an injury against the human spirit, and that could make them easier to control.

Severing that *natural relationship with food* also has profound social consequences, because food brings people together. The finding, preparing, and enjoying of food with others were communal activities that had always been a primary source of enrichment for human culture.

Doling out pre-made food that provided only bland, joyless sustenance will have gone some way to preventing slaves from forming those normal, empowering social bonds.

Yet another theory relates to the frequency of eating. We know that a carb-based diet requires more regular meals. This has also been documented in history, such as this account from the Mongols' conquest of the Chinese Jin Dynasty in the 13th century...

"The Chinese noted with surprise and disgust the ability of the Mongol warriors to survive on little food and water for long periods; according to one, the entire army could camp without a single puff of smoke since they needed no fires to cook.

Compared to the Jurched soldiers, the Mongols were much healthier and stronger. The Mongols consumed a steady diet of meat, milk, yogurt, and other dairy products, and they fought men who lived on gruel made from various grains. The grain diet of the peasant warriors stunted their bones, rotted their teeth, and left them weak and prone to disease. In contrast, the poorest Mongol soldier ate mostly protein, thereby giving him strong teeth and bones. Unlike the Jurched soldiers, who were dependent on a heavy carbohydrate diet, the Mongols could more easily go a day or two without food." ~ Jack Weatherford, Genghis Khan and the Making of the Modern World

Requiring frequent meals makes an individual more dependent on the source of that food. In the case of the slave, that is the Owner.

However, another biological factor may be relevant. Whenever you put food into your digestive system, it presents a challenge to the body, to which it must respond. We know that the pancreas will always send insulin into the bloodstream when you eat, but another hormone is also released.

The adrenal glands, which are attached to each kidney, always release the hormone *cortisol* after eating. That is the fight-or-flight signal, which makes us tense and ready for action. If our earliest ancestors evolved scavenging from predators' kills on the plains of Africa, it is possible that putting the body into a state of high alert when eating could be a helpful survival strategy.

Whatever the evolutionary reason, the more frequently you eat, the more cortisol the adrenal glands will release into the bloodstream. So eating constantly throughout the day, which of course is not our ancestral pattern, could leave you with an elevated residual level of stress hormone.

What's more, prolonged excess cortisol production eventually results in a state called *adrenal fatigue*, which can lead to low physical and mental energy, lack of motivation, and even depression. That would also make the slave more docile and less likely to stand up against their Owner.

Additionally, if an individual is dependent on carbs and does not get to eat frequently enough, that can cause elevated hunger signals and consequently yet more stress. So withholding food could also be used as a punishment and weapon of control.

We have seen there are many reasons why slave food helped the Owners to maintain dominance, by denying their slaves the opportunity to enjoy natural, healthy physical, mental, emotional, and communal well being.

We would hope that, over the centuries, our diets would improve along the path to more advanced civilization. Sadly, the reverse has proven to be the case.

In fact, all the factors that applied to slave food in ancient times are no less applicable today, for the simple reason that we are still slaves… better dressed and more comfortable ones, but slaves nonetheless. And food continues to be no less of a tool of domination.

The System is more all-encompassing than it ever was, and the System wants you to eat what's best for the System, not what's best for you! You easily can see what your role is in The System by seeing what you are given, and told, to eat.

If the practice of slavery—getting rich off the back of others' labor—was so profitable back then, why would the Owners ever give it up?

The answer is they wouldn't, and they didn't! Slavery never went away, it merely *evolved*.

Chapter 10:
Corporate Takeover

Civilized society is, in reality, a clever and elaborate theatrical show. Law and politics present a facade to distract the masses, giving the impression that things are being managed for the benefit of all.

In this grand show the actors are replaced and storylines recycled, while behind the scenes the ultimate objective has always been the Owners' relentless pursuit of more wealth and power.

The problem with the parasitical pursuit of wealth is that it can never be satisfied. It can only escalate.

Of course there is nothing *naturally* wrong with parasites. Within the greater cycle of life, parasites like mosquitoes still provide food for other creatures, and some intestinal worms can remove heavy metals from an animal's system. Of course any activity of parasites must always be bound into the great cycle of life by the balancing effect of nature's laws.

But, in inventing The System, mankind had created a structure whose thirst for more could never be quenched. By overlaying our own artificial rules on top of those natural laws, the System's rampant expansion could push forward unshackled.

Following the Pareto Principle and fuelled by the legalized occupation of farmland and slavery, cities had grown into states and states expanded into empires.

Continued technological advances such as bigger ships and gunpowder enabled the most advanced civilizations to compete for the acquisition of even more power, spreading across the world and plundering any and all resources they could find.

The British, Spanish, Dutch, French, and Portuguese all took to the high seas, racing to grab the remaining unclaimed land and to subjugate other "primitive" peoples into slavery.

By investing more heavily in ships and guns than its European competitors, the British Empire would become the greatest the world had ever seen. At its peak, Britain would rule over almost one third of the African population and one fifth of all the land on Earth, and prospered massively by bringing back all kinds of goods and treasure from the territories it conquered.

One natural commodity in particular drove fervent competition for land in the warmer regions of the world. Sugarcane originated in Asia where it had traditionally been chewed raw, however the invention of a process toextract sugar crystals, which would be easier to transport and did not spoil easily, happened in India around the third or fourth century CE.

Over the following centuries sugar spread eastwards and eventually reached Europe, where it was adopted with enthusiasm by the rich citizens, who grew particularly fond of adding it to two new luxury beverages, coffee and tea, which had recently arrived from the colonies.

The Europeans could not get enough of this product, but there were a couple of problems. Sugarcane would only grow in tropical climates, and its harvesting and processing was highly labor-intensive. That further fuelled the race to conquer more lands, including the Caribbean region, at the time dubbed "the sugar islands", as well as the need for many more slaves. It is estimated that up to twelve million slaves were transported from Africa to the Americas to provide manpower for the colonialists' projects.

By 1750, sugar had even overtaken grain as Europe's single most valuable traded commodity.

On the back of this wholesale colonization of land and humanity, Europe's wealth grew exponentially and, according to Pareto's abnormal model, so did its aspirations. With so much spare cash, overseas conquest projects became ever more ambitious until they outgrew the reach even of governments' tax coffers.

European superpowers needed a way to tap into the private resources of wealth held by rich landowners, but to do that would require the invention of a new type of legal structure that would allow the rich to pool their wealth to fund even more ambitious campaigns, while also limiting their individual risk.

The solution proved to be so useful for the Owners that it would eventually take over from conquest by nations using military force as the weapon of choice for domination. The invention of large *corporations*, operating within the fictional (i.e. bullshit) construct of international trade law, opened the door to take legalized theft and slavery truly global.

The idea of the *company* had existed for some time. A company made it possible for investors to join forces and to pool assets in order to do business jointly on a larger scale. In a company, the partners would be known to each other and they would also all share management responsibility, which meant ownership and control were inextricably linked.

However the fact that a company's owners were all personally liable constituted a limiting factor. As trading ambitions expanded, more capital would be needed, and that meant attracting money from a greater number of wealthy individuals.

The first corporations abstracted the concept of ownership by offering shares to investors. That meant the owners could now be anonymous and no longer involved in the day-to-day running of the business, which became the responsibility of its elected directors. That meant the owners were now *shielded from risk*, not only by limiting financial losses but also from any consequences arising from the actions of the corporation.

The earliest corporations had been set up to deliver specific, time-based, large projects, often in the public interest, such as building a canal or hospital. They were granted charters that would persist only for the set length of time needed to complete a project or voyage, usually no more than two or three decades, after which all the firm's holdings would be liquidated and any profits shared out among its investors.

At the turn of the seventeenth century, the prospect of trade with India and other territories required a whole new level of investment in shipping and manpower, as well as an increased need for military force, as the British, Dutch, and Portuguese in particular competed over the wealth of resources available in foreign lands.

That led to the creation of the first large corporations, such as we would recognize today, in the form of the British and Dutch East India Companies. Due to the great distances, the high risk, and the scale of work involved in long-term global trade projects, these corporations were granted longer charters. What's more, they were not required to return dividends immediately to investors but could hold profits in the business to fund further growth. Both corporations would go on to manage trade with the colonies, enjoying virtual monopolies, for the next hundred and fifty years.

For the first time, corporations were big enough to undertake massive, high-risk endeavors that would previously have been beyond the scope of groups of individuals, or even governments.

But it also meant we now had a situation where a corporation could operate freely with no comeback on its owners. The corporation is solely responsible for its own actions, liabilities, and debts while shareholders bear no personal liability whatsoever.

Corporations are novel *legal entities* in their own right. A corporation is termed an "artificial being" or "artificial person" in law, which means, for example, that it can sue or be sued in its own name. In fact, a corporation exists only "in contemplation of law". Outside of the law, a corporation literally *does not exist*.

Another important break away from nature is that, as a *non-living entity*, a corporation is *not capable* of moral agency. That means corporations can behave just like psychopaths because they truly *cannot care*.

The sole purpose of most corporations is to generate profits for its shareholders. In fact, its directors are usually obligated by a type of law called *fiduciary duty* to return the *maximum profits possible*.

In simple terms, using fictional corporations as vehicles for the acquisition of wealth now made the Owners literally untouchable! As history has shown time and again, it is possible to assassinate a monarch or a political leader, but it is impossible to kill a non-living corporation.

Even if a corporation does manage to get such a toxic reputation that it becomes too difficult to continue to trade, its assets can simply be sold to or merged with another corporation, allowing it effectively to be reborn and continue business as usual.

Now free from any moral responsibility, corporations offered the ideal cover and means for the spread of psychopathy through conquest and trade, adding yet more levels of anonymity and abstraction between the people of the world and the psychopaths who collect the profits.

Thanks to this new way of amassing wealth without responsibility, trade would soon prove to be even more profitable than overt military conquest, and corporations would soon become even more powerful than countries!

Over time, many occupied nations managed to organize uprisings and to regain their sovereignty from their invaders. The British Empire eventually figured out how to continue to dominate other nations without firing a shot, by establishing trading posts and the rule of law.

One example is the colonization of New Zealand, whose real name is Aotearoa. Wikipedia gives the following account:

"In 1840 the Treaty of Waitangi was signed between representatives of the United Kingdom and various Māori chiefs, bringing New Zealand into the British Empire and giving Māori the same rights as British subjects." (Wikipedia)

But history, as everyone knows, is written by the winners. The indigenous Māori would give a very different account. There had been in fact two treaties drawn up, one written in English legal language, the other in the native Māori tongue.

While there is much ongoing dispute, it appears the two documents differed significantly in content. The Māori never believed they were becoming subjects of the Crown, but were only allowing the British to trade through one port and set up one trading post.

However, after the document was signed, it was too late. The Māori discovered that they were now British subjects ("subject" literally means "to throw under") and prohibited from selling land to anyone but the British Government or its agents, leading to total occupation of the islands within a few generations.

This is one example of how the rule of law even allows governments and corporations to bind whole nations effectively into slavery, all done in plain sight, and proving the pen can indeed be mightier than the sword. (Of course, the sword never went away, because the law is always enforced by the looming threat of violence.)

"Lawyers can steal more money with a briefcase than a thousand men with guns and masks." ~ Don Vito Corleone, *The Godfather*

This can not even be called corruption. Provided a corporation acts in line with the objectives agreed at its foundation, and as long as contracts are agreed, it is all *legal*. It's not personal, just business. And of course the owners remain immune from any backlash.

In the mid-1700s the imperialistic East India Companies were finally dissolved, at the same time as innovations in coal power and engineering fueled a new era of growth as Britain and other countries entered the Industrial Revolution.

As machines enabled humans to extract more resources and produce more output, the Industrial Revolution ushered in a further dramatic change in the lifestyles and prospects of the masses.

While people had been using small-scale mechanization for centuries, such as grain mills powered by wind or water, the coal-powered steam engine meant those gave way to much larger mills and factories that could run constantly, twenty-four hours a day.

Such huge factories needed a constant supply of labor, which meant a static workforce was required. As most of the population still lived on the land at this time, the Owners needed a way to force large numbers to leave the countryside and move into towns so they could operate the machines.

The British Government issued a series of Acts of Enclosure, which reallocated most of the available farmland to new owners, thereby effectively prohibiting the traditional way of life in which villagers would be allowed to farm their surrounding fields. Taking away the people's ability to feed themselves forced mass migration into the towns.

The Owners also found a new way to keep the workforce in one place, by offering loans on housing: the mortgage (which literally means "death grip"). In order to feed themselves, and to cover their mortgage payments, the masses now depended on a regular wage from the mills and factories.

Forcing workers to endure extremely long working hours served as another weapon of control. A sixteen-hour working day was actually the norm in the Industrial Revolution… that's doing as much labor *in one day* that our Paleolithic ancestors needed to put in over a whole week!

Furthermore, the working poor still needed to feed themselves and their families, but having no spare time made self-sufficiency unthinkable. Never fear, the Owners were happy to ship food into the towns. Also, the cost of producing food, and grain in particular, had come down dramatically. Jethro Tull's invention of the seed drill in 1701 allowed seed to be planted automatically in the ground by a machine pulled behind a horse, proving far more efficient than previous human-powered broadcast methods.

Although the cost of producing grains dropped significantly, the new mechanical processes did not do much to make animal husbandry much more cost-efficient. As a result, grain-based foodstuffs like bread and porridge became the only staples the workers could afford. They would also have eaten on-site at factory canteens, giving us the now-standard three meals a day that happened to suit the industrial timetable.

We can see this new working class did not find themselves in a situation much different from the slaves of antiquity: they were also not free to move where they wished; they too were forced to work extremely long hours on menial and repetitive tasks; and of course, just like the slaves, they were given food that provided energy but without sufficient nutrition to keep body and mind in full health.

If such a life was little better than slavery, how could the owners get the working poor to put up with it? Here is where another new form of bullshit came in. Calvinism gave the people an extreme form of Protestant Christianity that held that the Scriptures were to be taken as literal truth and also preached the virtues of hard work and obedience. The new Protestant work ethic promised that suffering in this life would be rewarded in the next.

Of course it required significant investment to build a factory, so it was not an option for most people, but thanks to Pareto, those who had access to capital were able to multiply their wealth massively at this time.

If you were in a position to raise capital to build a factory, pay low wages, and churn out products far cheaper than could be done by traditional, artisan skills, the profits would follow, which allowed you to build more machines and factories, creating a positive feedback loop. Through this time of great innovation, thanks to the industrial economies of scale and a workforce that was enslaved, if not on paper but in practicality, the rich went on to make even greater fortunes, while the prospects of the poor remained miserable.

However, the Owners of the industrial age discovered that being able to mass-produce stuff with machines instead of skilled labor presented a brand new problem. If all you needed was the right machine, what would prevent another rich person from building a similar machine that could turn out the same product, maybe for an even lower cost?

That meant another type of new law was required to protect the intellectual property of inventions. While this may seem to make sense in the context of industrial design, of course it could never apply to the natural world. You could not, and still today cannot, patent something designed by nature, including natural foods.

However, as we will see, when industry and food production collided, and the new food industrialists needed to protect their investments in the same way, the health of the people would take yet another turn very much for the worse.

Chapter 11:
Factory Feed

Prior to the Industrial Revolution, food production was still predominantly a human, artisan activity. However the industrialists soon turned their attention to the food market, eyeing the opportunity for new profits made by applying the principles of the factory both to farming and to food manufacture.

The prime directive of most corporations is to maximize profits to the exclusion of moral questions. That means human and ecological health *cannot* factor in corporate decision making if they might get in the way of short-term profits.

The way to maximize profits is to make something at the lowest possible cost and to sell it at the highest price. Applying those principles to our food has come at a huge detriment both to humanity and to our environment.

In the realm of food production, the industrial requirement to keep costs to a minimum drove the invention of new, processed, agricultural commodities that possess features that are desirable to mechanized systems such as cheapness of production, standardization, ease of transport, and long shelf life.

Animals of course do not fit this model very well, as they are mobile and require more human intervention, but that has not stopped the food System from applying industrial methods to animals as far as it could. The result is confined feeding operations where cattle, poultry, and pigs are fed cheap, industrially-produced *feed* that is not species-appropriate.

In natural environments, all animals are free to move around, which means they are able instinctively to choose from a variety of food sources, enabling them to balance their nutrient requirements according to their bodies' signals and thereby maintain proper health.

When raising an animal only for slaughter, full health is of course not a major issue. In the System's view the beasts are nothing more than stock units. From the industrial mindset, all that is required is to get the animal to slaughter weight in a sellable condition as fast as possible. Animal feeds, supplements, and drugs have been developed over time to promote rapid growth and to accelerate fat gain.

We can all agree that the factory farming of animals is nothing short of an abomination against nature. But the changes to the human diet since it too became industrialized are having similar impacts on our own health prospects.

Factory farming of animals will never play a major part in the industrial food System because, when it comes to profit margins, it can never compare to the profitability of plant-derived commodities.

As we had discovered thousands of years previously, you can simply extract a lot more calories from good, arable land by growing crops than you can by raising animals. You do not get more nutrition, of course, and the whole process is fundamentally ecologically unsustainable, but the System does not care about these things.

Aside from the soil-killing action of the plow, creating monocultures, vast fields where just one single crop grows at a time, introduces a new set of problems. You never find monocultures in nature. Even grasslands, which might seem to be dominated by a single type of plant, are in fact extremely rich and diverse ecosystems, and that richness of life brings an inherent natural resilience. Everywhere in nature, complex colonies of plants, animals, fungi, and bacteria work in intricate harmony to maintain balance.

The monocultures you get with modern agriculture, on the other hand, are practically *ecological deserts*. Permitting only a single plant species to grow dramatically upsets the natural order.

On an industrial scale, weeding out undesirable plants by hand is not viable, which gave rise to chemical weed killers. Without the natural layers of defenses provided by nature's complex web of animal, fungal, and microbial life, monocrops are also far more vulnerable to being destroyed by pests, which in turn also led to the development of chemical pesticides.

Even with constant plowing and the mechanical application of chemicals to the land, and despite the occasional failed crop, agriculture continues to serve the System's needs very well, producing cheap commodity ingredients year after year, which can be sold at a healthy profit.

But the financial profit is the only aspect of this scenario that can be viewed as "healthy". Humans evolved eating plants only occasionally, and as such we lack the mechanisms to get all the nutrition we need from them.

The fact that plants cannot run away may be good for mechanization but it also has a serious impact on human health.

Consider that the only parts of any plant that are naturally *meant* to be eaten are fruits and nuts. Making fruits and nuts palatable is one of the mechanisms that plants use for spreading their genes to new places, along with other techniques such as wind dispersal of seeds.

Aside from that single biological imperative, plants have no interest in being eaten, therefore the vast majority have come up with defenses to discourage animals from consuming them.

Many plants are outright toxic or protected by thorns, but another very common defense is to create *antinutrients* that prevent the animal from being able to extract sufficient nutritional value, which means animals will quickly learn not to eat that particular plant.

As previously mentioned, any food we might ingest constitutes a challenge to the body. In fact, you might say that anything you ingest can be toxic to health. It is all a question of dosage.

Around five hundred years ago, the physician and chemist Paracelsus gave this basic principle of toxicology: "All things are poison and nothing is without poison; only the dose makes a thing not a poison." Even water and oxygen can be toxic to the human body in too great amounts or over too long a timeframe.

Now, the human body comes equipped with a marvelous variety of mechanisms to help us to deal with environmental toxins. We have the ability to excrete toxic substances via our livers and bowels, our kidneys and urine, and even through our breath, skin, and sweat. We can also store excess toxins in our fat cells for gradual, controlled release at a later time.

For our ancestors, eating a few grass seeds or fruits at the appropriate time of year was not a problem, as they could comfortably deal with any toxins in moderate amounts.

However, many of the plants we domesticated still retain a huge variety of toxins and antinutrients, which include tannins, oxalates, lectins, saponins, trypsin inhibitors, isoflavones, solanine, and chaconine.

But we are concerned most specifically with just a handful of plants, or their refined products, which very quickly came to form the *overwhelming majority* of what humans have consumed in the years following food industrialization.

Flour

Humans have been eating flour, most commonly in the form of bread, for millennia. Our consumption went up dramatically following the invention of new roller mill technology around 1880.

Refined flour is very high in starch, a carbohydrate, and there is no such thing as an essential carbohydrate in the human diet. Grains provide almost zero nutritional value, but do also contain a couple of notable antinutrients!

Phytic acid is an antinutrient found in both grains and legumes that interferes with the absorption of minerals, including phosphorus, calcium, copper, iron, magnesium, and zinc.

The other much more well known antinutrient is gluten. Gluten is a combination of two plant proteins, which is unusable by the human body, but causes significant damage to the gut, which can lead to leaky gut syndrome, systemic inflammation, allergic reactions, celiac disease, Crohn's disease, a range of autoimmune conditions, and even cognitive problems.

Throughout ancient times, the negative effects of gluten were mitigated by use of fermentation. Traditional breads all over the world were often made over several days using special yeasts, whose biochemical action would break down the gluten proteins into less harmful compounds.

Sugar

Refined sugar, extracted from tropical sugar cane, had also been around for many centuries, but the cost of production meant it was still a luxury item. Around 1800, a process was developed to extract sucrose from a new source, beets, which had the advantage of being able to grow in temperate climates. In 1822, the first industrial sugar extraction process was developed, and the first successful commercial production of beet sugar in the U.S. began in California in 1870.

The industrial processing of sugar beet led to a significant drop in the cost of production and consequently a rapid rise in usage.

Sugar is of course just pure refined carbohydrate. A sucrose molecule is actually one glucose molecule attached to a fructose molecule. These two molecules separate when sugar enters the bloodstream and *both* have antinutrient effects on the body.

The glucose molecule is very similar in structure to vitamin C (ascorbic acid). Both are transported across cell membranes into cells by insulin. Your entire bloodstream will normally contain no more than a teaspoonful of glucose, but higher concentration of glucose in the blood will compete with vitamin C transit, preventing it from getting where it needs to be in the cells.

In particular, leukocytes, which play a vital role in the immune system, require a large amount of vitamin C to operate effectively, eighty times the level normally present in the blood.

While most mammals can actually convert glucose into vitamin C, humans lack this ability, making it an *essential* nutrient that we can only get from our diets. However, the more sugar is consumed, the less efficiently our bodies are able to use vitamin C.

Ancestrally, we would only have encountered sugar in seasonal fruits and berries, or the occasional raid on a bees' nest. Plants put sugar in fruits *specifically* to make them appealing to animals. But it is important to note that natural fruits tend to be high in vitamin C as well! If plants only provided fruits with high sugar content but *without* a boost of extra vitamin C, gorging on fruit would make an animal, including a human, sick, so they would learn not to eat that fruit again.

The fructose molecule also causes problems in the body, driving the production of an enzyme that degrades stores of vitamin D, as well as interfering with another enzyme that helps with vitamin D production. Low vitamin D is a factor in poor immunity and many health issues, including cancers. Furthermore, vitamin D is also essential for calcium absorption, and excess sugar consumption not only makes it harder for the body to store the calcium it needs, but actually leads to more excretion of calcium, along with other essential minerals such as magnesium and chromium.

Corn

The corn plant has many similarities to wheat and other grains derived from annual grasses. It has been bred over the centuries to yield massive amounts of carbohydrates, which led to it becoming a highly profitable crop, yet again offers almost zero nutritional value.

Corn is less harmful than other grains in terms of antinutrients, as many can be removed by soaking, but it can contain fungal toxins (mycotoxins), which have been linked to issues with immunity, problems with the liver and lungs, as well as some cancers, if consumed excessively.

These three basic modern commodity crops offer very poor nutrition along with an abundance of unnecessary carbohydrates. However it is the fourth that has had by far the most profound negative impact on our health.

Seed Oils

We know that the Ancient Egyptians had extracted natural oils from seeds such as flax and linseed, which was surely a factor in their relatively high levels of chronic disease. However the process was labor-intensive and so seed oils would not constitute a large proportion of the general public's diet until the industrial era, when they would reemerge as a staple foodstuff and with disastrous consequences.

It is worth noting that prior to the twentieth century Americans consumed practically no seed oils. The first such product to be developed on an industrial scale was cottonseed oil, which was an unwanted by-product of the cotton industry.

Nobody could figure out how to extract the oil from the hard seeds efficiently until 1857 with the introduction of the first mechanical process. Cottonseed oil was originally used as fuel for oil lamps as well as an alternative to whale oil as a machine lubricant.

It was not considered as suitable for food use, not least because of its foul odor. It was only in 1899 when food chemist David Wesson found a way to deodorize it that cottonseed oil became a food product.

As it is made up of mostly (77%) unsaturated (i.e. unstable) fats, cottonseed oil is liquid at room temperature, making it more suitable for industrial processing than animal fats, which contain more saturated (stable) fatty acids and are therefore solid at room temperature, as liquids are easier and more cost-effective to move around with tankers, pumps, and pipes.

Two plucky entrepreneurs, William Procter and James Gamble, spied market opportunities for the new, cheap oil, which could be used in place of animal fats in the manufacture of candles, soap, and also *shortening*, replacing the lard, tallow, and butter that had traditionally been used in baking.

But that meant they had to find a way to make the oils solid. Unsaturated fats are unsaturated because some of the atoms in the carbon chain are missing hydrogen atoms. That means that one (in the case of monounsaturates) or more than one (polyunsaturates) pair of carbon atoms have double bonds with an adjacent carbon. And that in turn gives the fat molecules an irregular shape so they cannot stack close together in a solid block, making unsaturated fats liquid at room temperature.

To make seed oils behave like animal shortening, the scientists needed a way to force extra hydrogen atoms into the fatty acid molecules. With help from German chemist E. C. Kayser, they developed the process of *hydrogenation* thus creating the first industrial *trans fats*. In 1911 the new Procter and Gamble corporation offered the world the first "vegetable shortening", Crisco, which it presented as a healthier alternative to animal-based shortening, backed up with a massive marketing campaign based around a new Crisco cookbook, in which every recipe replaced the healthy animal fats with the new hydrogenated product.

In the years that followed, chemists and industrialists found new ways to extract edible oils from a range of other seeds including sunflower and safflower, as well as from other cheap products like rice bran and soybeans. Every one of these must go through a series of industrial processes to alter their smell and color, and to make them more resistant to oxidation.

Despite being industrially-manufactured products, they are all marketed as healthy-sounding "vegetable oils", despite the fact that not one of them is actually derived from a vegetable.

We now had a new type of foodstuff that was not only much cheaper to produce than animal fats, but that we were told was healthier too. The only problem is that they are not healthier, in fact they are downright toxic.

One of the major problems with seed oils comes from their proportions of omega-3 to omega-6 essential polyunsaturated fatty acids. These fatty acids are required for full health and the body cannot synthesize them efficiently, so we must get them from our diets.

When they are broken down in cells, omega-3 fats create compounds that have anti-inflammatory properties. The products of omega-6 fatty acids, on the other hand, are inflammatory, acting like an alarm mechanism to direct the immune system to clean up damaged cells.

One type of omega-6 acid plays a particular role in the fat storage cycle. *Linoleic acid* is the most common of the essential omega-6s. This fatty acid is vital to life, being present in all cell membranes, helping keep our skin, bones, and blood vessels healthy, and also playing a vital role in fertility.

Linoleic acid is present in small amounts in meat and fish all year round, but is found in far higher concentrations in nuts and seeds, which would only naturally be available for part of the year, high summer and autumn, which happens to be the time when animals store body fat for use as insulation and energy during the coming winter.

During that limited window, early humans would have had access to two key food elements together. The first is elevated amounts of omega-6 fatty acids which they would be getting from foraged nuts and seeds, or from the meat and fat of prey animals that had fed on grasses that had gone to seed. The other dietary component peculiar to this time of year would be excess sugars found in fruit and berries.

This particular combination of a spike in dietary omega-6 together with the rise in available carbohydrates was the key to helping our ancestors to survive the long, cold winter months, because together these two ingredients told their bodies to enter the critical "fat storage mode".

Of course, putting down body fat at that particular time of year was more important for the majority of our ancestors who lived at latitudes outside of the tropics, but the biological mechanisms still apply whatever your heritage.

When linoleic acid and sugars are both present in higher concentrations in the blood, that special combination signals to the body that it must be time to store fat for the winter ahead.

The extra sugar provides spare energy that can now be stored away. It causes elevated blood glucose levels, which trigger the pancreas to release insulin, causing an insulin spike.

Insulin does many jobs in the body, one of which is to instruct fat cells to lock into storage-only mode, ready to receive and store energy in the form of triglycerides. That also makes fat cells temporarily unable to release their stored fatty acids back into the bloodstream.

In addition to the effects of spiking insulin, consuming unsaturated fats also has a special role in accelerating fat storage.

When the body metabolizes saturated fats, a reaction takes place inside the mitochondria within fat cells, which release chemicals known as *reactive oxygen species* out into the host fat cell. The presence of those chemicals effectively signals to the fat cell that it is full, causing it to become temporarily resistant to insulin, which in turn means it stops absorbing any more triglycerides. As a consequence, more triglycerides remain in the bloodstream and that has the effect of making you feel satiated and no longer compelled to eat. This truth has been known for a long time.

"Fatty foods are crucial because they increase saticty and so decrease fat accumulation. Avoid sugar, sweets and potatoes, limit bread and vegetables. Meat of every kind may be eaten, and fat meat especially." ~ Ebstein, "Obesity and Its Treatment" (1882)

But unsaturated fats like linoleic acid are metabolized differently. When mitochondria break down either monounsaturated or polyunsaturated fats, fewer reactive oxygen species are released, and that means cells *remain responsive* to the effects of insulin. That in turn means extra triglycerides will continue to be pushed into cells, driving continued fat storage and also resulting in a more rapid drop back to low blood triglyceride concentration, which will trigger hunger signals.

We also know that some linoleic acid is converted into chemicals called endocannabinoids, which play a further role in suppressing satiation by stimulating the production of the hormone ghrelin whose role is to increase appetite. (In other words, seed oils give you the munchies!)

In summary, eating saturated fats leaves you feeling more satiated, but consuming unsaturated fats does the opposite, causing you to continue to feel hungry.

Understand that all these processes are good and make perfect sense in a natural, evolutionary context, when the body needs to store as much energy as possible as quickly as possible during the window of opportunity when food is very plentiful. So far, there is nothing wrong with this picture.

We need a certain amount of omega-6 fats in our diet, but remember also that *the dose makes the poison.*

Your body ideally can cope with a proportion of between one and five times the amount of omega-6 to omega-3 fatty acids, but the problem is that seed oils contain *far more* omega-6, and linoleic acid in particular!

Cottonseed oil delivers a massive 54:1, grape seed oil 74:1, while some sunflower oil can get close to 200:1! Anyone who consumes excess carbs *together with* excess omega-6 every day of the year will simply be in constant fat storage mode, as well as lacking in the full range of essential nutrients.

It is also important to note that human beings did not evolve on a diet in which grains were a major component. We are meant to get our omega-6 requirement from the meat and fat of the animals we hunted. Note that ruminant animals can actually convert omega-6 fats into other monounsaturated and saturated fats, which means that, in a natural environment, their fat will always have around an ideal 2:1 ratio of omega-6 to omega-3.

However, humans do not have the ability to do that conversion. In the human body, omega-6 fatty acids are used for structure and signaling. Because they would be present in small amounts in our diets, our bodies only know one thing to do with them: store them for later use. That means any excess omega-6s above the normal concentration will build up in our bodies over time, causing inflammation, obesity, and worse.

You might imagine that shifting to consuming so much omega-6 fat, combined with a diet high in carbohydrates but lacking in other nutrients would have a shockingly detrimental impact on human health.

It did!

Towards the end of the nineteenth century, a Canadian dentist called Weston A. Price became interested in the possibility that diet might be the primary factor in causing tooth decay. This question triggered a lifelong interest in the link between nutrition and disease.

Price noticed that, while infectious diseases were on the decline in the Western world at that time, more of the chronic health problems that were inflicting his patients, including dental caries (tooth decay), seemed to be *degenerative*. In other words people were somehow becoming feebler and sicker with each generation.

When he was unable to identify any kind of foreign matter, infection, or toxin that might be responsible, he hypothesized that the degeneration must be due to something that was *lacking*.

However, because he saw the same problems all around him in society, he had no control group against which to test his hypothesis, so he set off to find one. Crucially, this happened to be the same period when Western nations were starting to export their novel foodstuffs all around the world.

Price eventually traveled the whole world and came into contact with numerous tribes that had been living pre-industrial lifestyles and eating pre-industrial diets.

From the Eskimos (Inuit) of Canada to remote Swiss villages to Africa, the South Seas, and Australia, Price and his team of researchers painstakingly analyzed the dental, skeletal, and medical condition of thousands of subjects and made extensive notes, which he recorded in detail in his landmark 1939 book *Nutrition and Physical Degeneration*.

Time and again on these expeditions, Price was able to find individuals who were still following their traditional lifestyles as well as others from the exact same genetic lineage who had recently come into contact with the white man's diet, thus providing the controls that he needed. He was the first researcher to compare the before and after effects of the Western diet on subjects side-by-side.

His conclusions would and should shock any reader. After even one generation consuming a Westernized diet, Price repeatedly observed the manifestation of physical deformities. The same patterns appeared over and over again, in every group he surveyed, from every corner of the Earth. His initial concern was in dental caries, and that certainly exploded after the introduction of modern foodstuffs, going from affecting typically between zero and two percent of the teeth observed up to fifty percent or more.

But, even more concerning, he discovered other patterns: narrowing of the face, smaller nostrils leading to mouth-breathing, crowding of teeth, all *within a single generation* of being exposed to Western food, or when a child's mother had been in the first generation. He even observed a consistent correlation between dental caries and tuberculosis.

Price's conclusion was that a lack of vital nutrition, in particular fat-soluble vitamins, must be the direct cause of this rapid physical degeneration. In fact, later tests with his own patients showed that tooth decay could actually be prevented with the supplementation of cod liver oil and high quality butter, which suggests that, *even if sugar in the diet does stimulate caries*, the body can still prevent it if sufficiently nourished with fat-soluble vitamins.

Price's discoveries extended beyond solely physical degeneration. He also noticed other consistent patterns: the physically most robust peoples also seemed to be healthier mentally, morally, and socially.

The consistency of the cause-and-effect pattern that Price observed first-hand provides indisputable proof that an innutritious diet rapidly degrades the human condition, causing what have been called "diseases of civilization". He wrote:

"Almost everyone who studies the matter will be surprised that such clear-cut evidence of a decline in modern reproductive efficiency could be all about us and not have been previously noted and reviewed."

He also dared to raise the obvious question of social ethics:

"Is it just for society to permit production of physical and mental cripples?"

Back in 1939 we had incontrovertible proof of the terrible consequences of a diet based on industrially-produced commodities. Like Price, we should all ask why nothing has been done to reverse the situation... but sadly we already know the answer.

There is far more profit in industrial food than in real food, and the corporate-run System is bound to push us to consume what is most profitable, paying no mind to any consequences such as long-term health.

In this way, can we say that the products of the industrial human food System are any better than what is given to animals on factory farms? Is the population considered any different to livestock? Is the food that we are being sold even "food" at all... or should we consider it nothing more than "feed"?

Factory feed had become the new slave food. But the System was not done yet, not while there were more profits to be made. Things were about to get even worse for humanity, powered by a whole new level of bullshit.

Chapter 12:
Science Fiction

If Weston Price proved beyond all doubt that the modern industrial diet was literally degrading humanity, it is reasonable to think the powers that be would be swift to do something about the problem.

But, rather than turn things around, the System proceeded to double down on its quest for profit, and in the process also accelerated the destruction of both human health and the earth beneath our feet.

In fact, Price is just one of many outliers that have been sounding the alarm over and over across the generations. The evidence has always been right there in plain sight in the public domain, because it could not be concealed without breaking the illusion.

A tiny minority of Owners cannot possibly control the vast majority through totalitarian domination alone. It is crucial that society continue to *appear to be run* in the interests of all. That's why they cannot completely block out free speech or free, true science.

But they do have their secret weapon: bullshit of various forms including the political pantomime and the mainstream media. That means the Owners have significant power to control what the masses *hear*.

In this chapter, we will see how the System has continually suppressed the voices of those outliers who dared to share any facts that do not support its goals, and given airtime to "alternative facts" that do.

Everyone knows that eating meat, and particularly saturated fat, is bad for your health... right?

Nope, of course that is a myth, which was fabricated in the middle of the last century to protect the profits of the industrial feed System. In fact, just about everything they've told you about how to eat healthily is pretty much the opposite of the truth!

Today it is easy to see that obesity and chronic conditions like heart disease and cancer now afflict the majority of the West, and rapidly increasing numbers in the rest of the world. It might seem bizarre to contemplate but, prior to the twentieth century, these conditions were *extremely rare*.

Fortunately, researchers have been able to uncover some historical records that throw the modern health crisis into stark contrast.

Data recorded on the weights and heights of male prisoners held in Texas and Nebraska prisons in the early 19th century show that, using today's BMI measurements, only just over one in a hundred (1.2%) would be categorized as obese. Within two centuries, that figure would balloon to close to half the US population.

In 2011 a report was published using historical records that listed the cause of every death that occurred in the town of Boston in the year 1811, offering a rare insight into what was killing people two centuries ago. The Boston report recorded only 5 out of 942 deaths from cancer, that's around one in two hundred. Today, we are told that *half* of us will suffer from cancer in our lifetimes.

The Boston report also documented *zero* deaths from heart attacks, although 2.6% of deaths were listed as "sudden death". It is extremely unlikely that these were caused by heart disease when you consider that throughout the entire nineteenth century there were only *eight* reports of heart attacks *worldwide*, and that the first heart attack in the United States would not be recorded from autopsy until 1912.

But, even if we assume that *all* these deaths were a result of heart disease, that still only accounts for one in forty deaths. In the present day, coronary heart disease is the single biggest killer in the United States, responsible for almost *one in four* of all deaths.

We can see that, within the space of just a few generations, obesity, cancer, and heart disease exploded from marginal issues into their current *epidemic proportions*. Of course we should ask why, what changed, and what has been done to turn the situation around.

Sadly, the real answers to these questions have been deliberately and systematically suppressed in favor of misleading fakery, with devastating, deadly consequences.

Even as early as the 1860s, an English carpenter William Banting had published his booklet *Letter on Corpulence*, which expounded the benefits of a high-fat diet for health and weight loss. Banting's diet philosophy would later be confirmed by Weston Price and many others.

"I can confidently state that quantity of diet may safely be left to the natural appetite; and that it is quality only which is essential to abate and cure corpulence."

In 1869, doctor Thomas Hawkes Tanner's book *The Practice of Medicine* explained the link between refined carbohydrates and weight gain, "Farinaceous and vegetable foods are fattening, and saccharine matters are especially so."

Another outlier Vilhjalmur Stefansson was an Icelandic-born American explorer who led a number of extended expeditions into the Canadian Arctic between 1906 and 1918. On one of his early trips north, when a ship carrying supplies failed to arrive, Stefansson was forced to live on the all-meat diet of the local Inuit people.

Already by that time, the general consensus on diet was that eating too much meat would lead to serious health problems, including rheumatism, hardening of the arteries, high blood pressure, and kidney damage.

However, after a decade of living almost continuously among the Inuit, Stefansson experienced none of these issues, but rather found his health *improved* on their high-animal-fat diet. He came to realize that everything he had been taught about nutrition and dietetics must be wrong, and would go on to be a vocal advocate for a high-fat, all-meat diet for the rest of his life.

Upon their return to the United States, Stefansson and a colleague volunteered to participate in an experiment at Bellevue Hospital, which involved consuming meat and fat exclusively for a full year under medical supervision. The results of the experiment that were published in the Journal of Biological Chemistry in February 1930 concluded that the men were both in fine health, mentally alert, with ideal blood pressure and free from any deficiencies, lending weight to Stefansson's assertion that it is perfectly possible for the body to meet all its nutritional needs from meat and fat alone.

Of course the majority of the population have never heard of this experiment or of Vilhjalmur Stefansson. If you check his Wikipedia entry, you will see how history (which of course is written by the winners) would prefer him to be remembered.

When coronary heart disease started to emerge as a major cause of premature death in the 1920s, the issue was not seen as an urgent priority. At this time, following the First World War, the US government was primarily concerned with ensuring people got enough to eat. Also, the nutritional content of food had never been an issue before.

Aside from heart disease, the twenties also saw the expansion of new types of bullshit in the form of advertising and public relations. Prior to that time, advertising had been a straightforward, mainly factual communication of a product and its benefits. But a new protagonist would apply recent developments in psychology to give the System another very powerful tool of control.

Edward Bernays was the nephew of Sigmund Freud, acknowledged as the father of psychology. Very much in the spirit of Machiavelli four centuries earlier, Bernays showed American corporations how his uncle's work could be adapted into a tool of mass manipulation. He developed techniques for persuading the people to buy things they did not need by linking them to subconscious desires. As his Wikipedia entry illustrates,

"Bernays described the masses as irrational and subject to herd instinct—and outlined how skilled practitioners could use crowd psychology and psychoanalysis to control them in desirable ways."

Bernays gives the following overview of how the techniques work in his 1928 manual *Propaganda*.

"Universal literacy was supposed to educate the common man to control his environment. Once he could read and write he would have a mind fit to rule. So ran the democratic doctrine. But instead of a mind, universal literacy has given him rubber stamps, rubber stamps inked with advertising slogans, with editorials, with published scientific data, with the trivialities of the tabloids and the platitudes of history, but quite innocent of original thought."

He also provided a rare description of how the Owners operate behind the cover of politics.

"There are invisible rulers who control the destinies of millions. It is not generally realized to what extent the words and actions of our most influential public men are dictated by shrewd persons operating behind the scenes."

One of Bernays' most infamous campaigns was a 1929 effort to get more women to smoke by branding cigarettes as feminist, labeling them "Torches of Freedom". He is also credited for inventing the concept of breakfast cereal, helping to create a lucrative new market for the United States' glut of grains.

"The [First] World War and the following inflation pushed the price of wheat to new high levels and caused a remarkable extension of the area planted to this crop. When the price collapsed during the post-war period Great Plains farmers continued to plant large wheat acreages in a desperate endeavor to get money with which to pay debt charges, taxes, and other unavoidable expenses. They had no choice in the matter." ~ Great Plains Committee, 1936

In the 1930s, the U.S. experienced the first warning signs that the very foundation of its agricultural economy could be in jeopardy. Following the wide scale adoption of petroleum-powered farm machinery, the fertile soils of the Midwest, which the first European settlers had reported as being several feet deep, had already degraded into dirt, leading to the "Dust Bowl" and causing general alarm.

"I suspect that when people along the seaboard of the eastern United States began to taste fresh soil from the plains 2,000 miles away, many of them realized for the first time that somewhere something had gone wrong with the land." ~ Hugh Bennet, Soil Conservation Chief, 1941

As the desire for cheap commodity crops proceeded to expand, the soil would only continue to deteriorate, and along with it the nation's health.

But global politics and economics would only further drive the development of factory-produced processed foods.

In the Second World War, the U.S. military needed a reliable way to get calories to men fighting all around the world. That need drove the development of a range of new methods of processing and preservation.

In 1941, an ambitious physiologist from the University of Minnesota named Ancel Keys was charged with creating a pocket-sized, non-perishable ration pack that could keep combatants going in the field. His final product was based on highly processed items with long shelf life, such as hard biscuits, canned processed meat, candy, and chocolate.

Test subjects described the ration pack—which would go on to be known as the "K ration"—as "palatable" and "better than nothing", but it achieved the objective of getting calories into the troops reliably... and cheaply.

After the war ended, advertising helped to ensure that the methods and processing facilities that produced the K ration would continue to have a purpose. As more women went out to work, the marketing sector told them that cooking equated to drudgery and now "convenience" became a new buzzword that represented emancipation, in the process giving the world new ways to eat such as freeze-dried mashed potato and oven-ready TV meals.

By 1940, coronary heart disease had taken over as the single leading cause of death in the United States, so scientists turned their attention to the search for a cause.

In the late 1940s, research doctor John Gofman discovered and categorized different types of lipoprotein (commonly referred to as "cholesterol") particles in blood. Several decades before, in the 1910s, a German chemist Adolph Windaus had noticed the presence of cholesterol in atherosclerosis, arterial plaque deposits. Around the same time, another scientist, the Russian Nikolai Anitschkow, had fed rabbits (who are of course obligate herbivores) a mixture of cholesterol and sunflower oil, and noticed that they developed a form of atherosclerosis.

Gofman went on to speculate that it was cholesterol particles that *caused* the atherosclerosis and that it could also go on to cause other health issues such as coronary heart disease. However, it would not be Gofman who built a career on these ideas, which would come to be known as the Diet-Heart Hypothesis.

At the time heart disease was emerging as the major public health concern, it was in fact Ancel Keys who picked up on Gofman's ideas and became obsessed with proving that cholesterol must somehow be to blame. He was determined to be seen by the public as a savior and devoted himself to this cause.

Fuelled by immense self-belief, charisma, and ruthless determination, Keys helped to bring about the emergence of a major new force in U.S. health research with the backing of a powerful corporate sponsor.

In 1948, Procter and Gamble, maker of the vegetable oil-based shortening Crisco, sponsored a radio contest that raised $1.7 million on behalf of a small, cash-strapped group of health professionals known as the American Heart Association. The sponsorship quickly catapulted the AHA from a minor special interest society into the country's largest nonprofit organization.

It is interesting to note that the AHA would go on to invest hundreds of millions of dollars into research, with the primary aim of promoting public acceptance of the Diet-Heart Hypothesis that Ancel Keys touted as his own.

Keys initially spent years trying to prove a link between dietary cholesterol and coronary heart disease, but no matter how much cholesterol he fed to human subjects, no impact on their serum levels could be observed and he was forced to admit that...

"The evidence – both from experiments and from field surveys – indicates that cholesterol content, per se, of all natural diets has no significant effect on either the cholesterol level or the development of atherosclerosis in man."

In the quest for a new research angle, Keys happened upon a document from the World Health Organization that seemed to suggest a possible association between dietary fat intake and heart disease deaths in twenty-two countries, with the United States topping the list for mortality.

In 1953 Keys presented this data at a WHO seminar but his methods were publicly criticized by two doctors who quite rightly pointed out that association does not imply causation.

Another problem was that Keys had cheated. Later analysis proved that, out of the original set of twenty-two countries, he had deliberately cherry-picked only a handful that would provide results that fit his final desired graph suggesting a causal relationship, and excluded any, including Switzerland, France, and Chile, all of which have both high dietary fat consumption and low heart disease rates, and whose inclusion would have proved there was in fact no statistically-relevant correlation.

The philosopher Karl Popper describes the attitude of a true scientist as being imbued with a "ruthless skepticism toward your own work". Ancel Keys was clearly never imbued with that trait. On the contrary, a proud and vain man, Keys took the chastisement personally and, rather than commit to seeking the truth, became even more determined to vindicate his ideas in the eyes of the world.

The profile of the heart disease epidemic was further thrust into the national spotlight when in 1955 President Dwight Eisenhower suffered the first of several heart attacks. The country was clamoring for answers, and of course Keys was more than happy to step up to the plate.

With presidential approval and funding from the U.S. Public Health Service, he went on to follow up on the WHO report with his own "Seven Countries Study", which would run from 1958 to 1980. The project involved interviewing over twelve thousand men in different countries and mapping the number of heart attacks experienced against dietary fat intake.

Keys published early results from the study that he claimed showed a clear correlation between fat consumption and heart attack rates, leading him to announce that:

"Whether or not cholesterol etc., are involved, it must be concluded that dietary fat somehow is associated with cardiac disease mortality, at least in middle age."

In fact the Seven Countries Study proved no such link between dietary saturated fat and heart disease. But it would not matter.

The world now had what it craved: a simple answer. All you had to do was remove saturated fat and Keys said the problem of coronary heart disease would "become very rare". By now Ancel Keys was established as a celebrity scientist, even going on to appear on the cover of Time magazine in January 1961.

Perhaps the fact that his conclusions happened to suit very nicely the objectives of the industrial processed feed sector, which specializes in producing cheap commodity ingredients from large-scale farming of plants is the real reason why his unfounded proclamations continued to dominate health advice, and do so even up to the present day.

"The only sure way to control cholesterol is to reduce fat in the U.S. diet from 40% to 15% of total calories and cut saturated fats from 17% to 4% of total calories... Americans eat too much fat and most of that is saturated which damages arteries and leads to coronary artery disease."

In another example of Keys' sleight-of-hand, many such references to "saturated" fats in his experiments, which he *implied* come from natural sources like eggs and butter, were actually artificial trans fats from industrially-hydrogenated seed oil products such as margarine.

Because Keys, and the food System that supported him (including secret financial backing from the sugar industry), suppressed those facts, it would not be until 1978 that trans fats would finally be proven to have a multitude of toxic effects, including leading to fatty liver disease, obesity, heart attacks, and strokes, forcing Procter and Gamble to reformulate their Crisco vegetable shortening.

What's more, as part of the Seven Countries Study, Keys had also compiled data on the role of smoking in heart disease, but he failed to publish those findings, which *did* show a clear correlation, until 1980!

As a result of the corporate-sponsored demonization of animal fats, by the end of the 1950s, the obesity rate had climbed to 13% and the average American now carried 9.1% linoleic acid in their body fat.

Aside from Vilhjalmur Stefansson's results from twenty years earlier, many other voices continued to discover, and to advocate for, the health benefits of fatty meat.

In 1949 a paper had reported the results of a program in which twenty executives of the Dupont corporation, all described as obese, were put on a strict diet of three parts meat to one part fat. Even though the participants were allowed to eat as much as they liked, the results showed that, over periods ranging from six weeks to six months, they lost on average 22 pounds, their blood pressure dropped, and they reported enjoying increased energy levels and confidence.

In 1950, Elizabeth Woody published an article "Eat all you want reducing diet" in Holiday magazine that allowed for unlimited meat and fat.

In 1957, a doctor called George Thorpe also advised that obese patients who wanted to lose weight must follow a high-protein, high-fat, low-carbohydrate diet.

Yet the mainstream narrative continued to parrot Ancel Keys' phony assertions that placed the blame on animal fats, while deflecting attention away from the real culprits: seed oils, refined carbohydrates, and sugar.

There are countless more examples that show how corporate cash manipulated the scientific narrative over the coming decades.

For his 1957 book *A History of Nutrition*, Professor E. V. McCollum of Johns Hopkins University published the summary of his survey of 200,000 scientific papers reporting on the results of nutrition experiments that had been published between 1816 and 1940.

Bizarrely, *A History of Nutrition* did not include a single experiment that looked at sugar! However, the book's introduction includes the following words:

"The author and publishers are indebted to The Nutrition Foundation, Inc., for a grant provided to meet a portion of the cost of publication of this book"

Who or what is "The Nutrition Foundation"? It turns out to be a conglomerate of about forty-five processed food manufacturers including the American Sugar Refining Company, Coca-Cola, Pepsi-Cola, Curtis Candy, General Foods, General Mills, and Nestlé.

In 1958, Time magazine printed an article reporting that a biochemist at Harvard University, with sponsorship from the Sugar Research Foundation, had spent ten years researching interventions that might prevent sugar from causing dental caries. After countless experiments on mice, the researchers reported that they had been able to come up with no way to prevent tooth decay, and found that their funding was immediately withdrawn.

Time and time again, many expensive and large-scale trials would consistently fail to provide proof to support Keys' hypothesis.

In 1968, an intervention trial was run with 846 middle-aged men in a Los Angeles hospital for veterans that would track the effects of replacing saturated fats with hydrogenated polyunsaturated vegetable oils. No improvement was found in overall mortality, although cancer rates *did* increase in the intervention group who had been given the industrial fats.

Another experiment, the New York Diet and Coronary Heart Disease study led by Norman Jolliffe MD, which ran from 1957 to 1972, found *more* deaths in the randomized group that had been given polyunsaturated fatty acid-enriched margarines and "vegetable" oils in place of animal fats. The authors did their best to cover up that particular evidence.

The Framingham Heart Study, which was one of the most robust studies of its kind, ran for thirty years from 1948. It *did* find some correlation between high cholesterol levels and coronary heart disease. However it also found that the group with higher cholesterol also happened to live longer, while those with lower cholesterol were at increased risk of developing cancer. Ultimately, the study concluded that, for each one percent *drop* in serum cholesterol, there was a corresponding eleven percent *increase* in mortality! As a consequence, no report of these findings was published. The truth was only later disclosed by one of the members of the study group, George Mann MD, who had resigned when he became aware of the subterfuge.

Between 1968 and 1973, Ancel Keys himself ran what was, on this occasion, a perfectly designed and executed study. The Minnesota Coronary Experiment (MCE) was a large-scale, double-blind, randomized controlled trial on over 9000 test subjects in seven different institutions. When the experiment conclusively disproved the Diet-Heart Hypothesis, true to form, Keys buried the findings, which would remain unpublished until 1989.

Between them, the MCE and two other large scale randomized controlled trials, the Women's Health Initiative Randomized Controlled Dietary Modification Trial and the

Sydney Diet Heart Study, would rack up total costs approaching *one billion U.S. dollars.*

Tim Noakes, professor at the University of Cape Town and distinguished member of the National Research Council, explains that, far from proving any health benefit from replacing saturated fats with unsaturated fats, these gold-standard trials have unequivocally established that removing saturated fat from the diet actually has the *opposite* effect.

"The tragedy was that, hidden in the data, was the evidence that the diet caused harm. That re-analysis by independent scientists established that removing saturated fat from the diet to lower the blood cholesterol concentrations caused measurable harm, especially to those with pre-existing heart diseases or type 2 diabetes mellitus, more so in those over 65 years of age."

"So powerful is this evidence that, in my opinion, it should be the end of the debate."

In fact, the most significant insight so far discovered in predicting coronary heart disease risk is that a *higher concentration* of HDL-cholesterol in the blood leads to *lower risk.* While this should be the final nail in the coffin of the Diet-Heart hypothesis, it remains a little-publicized fact.

In 1971 the Honolulu Heart Study found only one statistically significant correlation: that cutting dietary carbohydrates reduced the incidence of heart disease.

In 1972 John Yudkin, a British nutritionist and former Chair of Nutrition at Queen Elizabeth College, London, published his book *Pure, White and Deadly*, which explored the health risks of sugar in the diet, to a storm of criticism and ridicule from the sugar industry, manufacturers of processed foods, as well as from Ancel Keys. Yudkin and Keys had a long-running feud, with one seeking to place the blame for heart disease on sugar, the other on fat. Neither was able to produce sufficient evidence, for the reason that the relationship between nutrition and health is far too complicated to implicate one single macronutrient. (In fact, the best single indicator for predicting heart disease is really *affluence*: the more food available to a population, the higher the risk.)

We have only mentioned a fraction of the studies that prove the Diet-Heart hypothesis to be comprehensively and conclusively wrong. So, with decades of scientific research that points diametrically in the other direction, why does the blame continue to be laid at the door of saturated fat?

It is just the way the System works. Even if it means flying in the face of the increasing weight of evidence, the System *must* pursue whatever courses of action generate the maximum profits for the Owners.

By 1980, one in five American adults would already be obese, heart disease and cancer rates were still rocketing skyward... but the Owners were not done yet!

Now that "everybody knew" that animal fats were unhealthy and plant-based alternatives were preferable, the System had yet another trick up its sleeve to persuade the masses to consume even more cheap, industrially-produced feed.

All that was needed was yet another, even more wide-reaching layer of bullshit.

Chapter 13:
The Food Education Industry

The very concept that we need to be told by strangers what to put in our mouths is extremely recent, and, like everything else that the System abstracts to take us further away from our natural way of living, is open to abuse. As we will see in this chapter, today's dietary guidelines, while purporting to support the nation's health, are nothing more than bullshit corporate propaganda.

Governments only started to give people dietary advice very recently, in the twentieth century. The first policies focused on ensuring people were eating *enough*, but with the discovery of vitamins and essential minerals and the increasing prevalence of chronic disease, the focus shifted to nutrition.

Have you ever wondered why we should have to be told what to eat at all? We are supposedly the most intelligent species on Earth yet also the *only* creature that lacks the ability even to figure out how to meet its most basic biological needs!

For the vast majority of our time here, just like every other living thing, humans simply went out and got the food they needed from nature. Long ago our ancestors learned from experience what was good and what was harmful and passed that knowledge on to each subsequent generation.

That started to change when the Neolithic Agricultural Revolution and the shift from extensive to intensive living introduced new sources of food and the majority came to depend on others for their sustenance. When you look back over history, you see a clear pattern of increasing intensification, the concentration of power and control into ever-fewer hands. What started with the control of food supply extended to the control of information, and now even the question of what to eat has been intensified into the control of an elite few.

Today, we have been duped into accepting the ludicrous concept that it is the job of government to tell us how to be healthy. The only reason it seems to make any sense to us that a bunch of rich men should tell us what to eat is because we have been indoctrinated to obey authority since preschool, as Denise Minger writes in her book *Death By Food Pyramid*.

"The reality is that most of us grow up strapped in an educational system that favors obedience over independent thinking. We're rewarded for trusting authority, and punished for challenging it."

It is easy to show that governments do not care either about saving lives or ending hunger when you consider that ten million people die of starvation every year. It would cost no more than around one thousand dollars to spare each soul, giving a total bill of ten billion dollars to put an end to world hunger. The U.S. military budget for 2022 was $715 billion, so we can close that line of inquiry and move on.

The fact that knowing what and how to eat is *no longer intrinsic* is the result of perhaps the biggest—and most harmful—scam ever perpetrated on the human race.

The next absurdity to highlight is that the primary source of Americans' dietary advice is the US Department of Agriculture, which has been responsible for publishing national dietary guidelines for decades. The USDA is *literally* the branch of government responsible for representing the interests of the country's growers. How can it possibly do that while also prioritizing the nation's health?

The picture starts to make more sense when you realize how much money is moving around. The US Government introduced farm subsidies back in the 1930s to help ensure the continuity of the nation's food supply in the Great Depression. At that time, thirty million Americans lived and worked on more than six million farms.

The practice of subsidies continues to this day, although now there are only about 3.4 million farmers, almost a tenth of the workforce a century ago. Nevertheless, with modern agricultural technology, American farms generated sales topping $350 billion in 2020, of which $192 billion came from plant crops, which surely makes the farming lobby a major force in domestic politics.

How much is paid out in subsidies? A stunning $25 billion of taxpayers' money every year. You may not be surprised to discover that more than seventy percent of that cash is handed out to growers of just three cheap commodity row crops: wheat, corn, and soybeans.

In reality it is not even those who grow the crops that ultimately benefit the most. As long as subsidies help to keep production costs down, the real beneficiaries are the corporate, industrial feed manufacturers who transport those taxpayer-subsidized ingredients to factories to be turned into *ultra-processed* products for sale to the consumer.

Humans have always used a variety of processes to make our food go further, such as curing, smoking, pickling, and fermenting. Traditional basic items like cheese and bacon are processed foods. It is vital to appreciate that today's *ultra-processed* products are very different. These are novel, artificial inventions that are reconstructed from simple commodity ingredients and churned out by massive industrial production lines.

As we have seen, the industrial system can only work efficiently with certain types of basic materials, those which come in standardized, small, easily transportable forms that will move smoothly through machinery. That's why the preferred ingredients are corn, soy, wheat, seed oils, and sugar, along with their numerous derivatives including high-fructose corn syrup and soy protein isolate.

Modern, industrial farming is huge business, and the biggest profits come from the cheapest crops, with corn generating $46 billion and soy $36 billion in sales annually. But all that is dwarfed by the American packaged food market, which turns over *one trillion* dollars per year.

As the department responsible for this enormous industry is also the one that tells Americans what they should be eating, surely there is bound to be a massive conflict of interest. One woman's story, as Denise Minger relates in *Death by Food Pyramid*, provides all the proof you need.

In the 1970s, the USDA hired a group of nutritionists to draw up the nation's next food guide, which would replace the "Basic Four" food groups that had been around since the mid-fifties.

The team, headed by Luise Light who was passionately committed to public health, proceeded to scour all the available literature to discover the latest and best science connecting diet with health, which led to the *first ever* set of recommendations that had been designed specifically to tackle the problem of chronic disease. The team's evidence-based recommendations put the focus on fresh produce, capped sugar intake to no more than ten percent of total calories, and set a maximum limit of two or three daily servings of grains.

The guide was duly submitted to the USDA for approval, but when it came back, it was unrecognizable! For example, the grain allowance had swelled back up to a massive *eleven daily servings*. What's more, the strict sugar limit had been softened to the vague word "moderate".

Again we must stress that this is not corruption, it's just business. The USDA is just doing what it has to do to fulfill its responsibility to America's farmers, and to the enormous corporations that buy their crops.

The same pattern continues to be evident wherever you look. For example, the latest US guide, "MyPlate", proclaims...

"It's important to eat a variety of fruits, vegetables, grains, protein foods, and dairy and fortified soy alternatives. When deciding what to eat or drink, choose options that are full of nutrients. Make every bite count."

Yet the guide fundamentally contradicts itself because it also recommends around a *third* of your diet should come from grains, which of course provide practically *zero* nutritional value, never mind all the antinutrients!

Or take the UK's current "Eatwell" guide, which also recommends about a third of the diet should be made up of grains, while recommending eating "less red meat" and "more beans and pulses". Perhaps the picture becomes clearer when you realize the committee that designed that guide included representatives from Kellogg's, Coca-Cola, British Sugar, McDonald's, and Starbucks among many other makers and retailers of ultra-processed products.

The team behind the 2017 EAT Lancet guide also reads like a who's who of large corporate interests, including Cargill, PepsiCo, Unilever, Nestlé, and—again—Kellogg's. No surprise then that it includes allowances for cakes, candy, chocolate, potato chips, soda, and ice cream as part of a "healthy" diet. In fact, an analysis of the total macronutrients in the diet the guide recommends shows it would actually deliver *more* calories from sugar than from meat!

The results are in. Your dietary advice does not come from science, nor even from the government, but from the corporations that make and sell ultra-processed grocery products.

The mainstream narrative continues to repeat unfounded claims that date all the way back to Ancel Keys' ideas from the 1950s, which have been disproven at every turn, while voices that proclaim factual evidence continue to be denied airtime.

For example the joint US-German study published in 2012 that showed that dairy fat intake resulted in *less* heart disease and type-2 diabetes...

Or a study from Queensland, Australia in 2016 that showed that drinking full-fat milk *lowered* the risk of heart attack by sixty percent...

Or the *Pure Study*, published in 2017 that surveyed 135,000 men and women in eighteen countries and concluded there was no correlation between saturated fat in the diet and either coronary heart disease or increased mortality. (It did, however, find that those who ate more saturated fat had a *reduced* incidence of stroke...)

Or how about a report published in 2017 in the British Journal of Sports Medicine that concluded that saturated fat does not clog arteries, but rather that coronary heart disease is actually a *chronic inflammatory condition*?

We might ask why it is even necessary to continue to explore the scientific dead-end that is the relationship of saturated fat to heart health, but we should certainly wonder why the flood of negative results continues to be suppressed in favor of the Keysian myth!

Another notable outlier, who undertook the task of collating *all* the evidence, is Dr. Zoë Harcombe. After taking redundancy from her previous career in management, Zoë was in the privileged position of being free to choose her own Ph.D topic, without the need for the corporate or government sponsorship that is a requirement for the vast majority of high-level research today.

Harcombe decided to turn her prodigious analytical skills to the problem of the obesity epidemic and specifically to see how closely it was based on the available *actual science.*

Her first conclusion was that we did not get fat because we were eating any more than previous generations, nor were we moving less. Ultimately, the only possible source for the obesity epidemic had to have come from *the dietary guidelines themselves*, as the rate of obesity accelerated immediately after their introduction and continues on the same trajectory. (Meanwhile in the United States another outlier, Gary Taubes, was coming to the same conclusions for the American population.)

For her Ph.D thesis, published in 2016, Harcombe undertook an exhaustive, systematic review of *all* the scientific evidence that had been available at the time the national dietary guidelines were introduced, in 1977 in the US, and 1983 in the UK.

Her conclusion: Based on the science, dietary fat guidelines should *never* have been introduced. Her later research, brought up to date with all the current science available today, also proved that there is no more evidence to support the national dietary guidelines now than there was a few decades ago.

She proved beyond all doubt that the total evidence to support the hypothesis that eating meat or fat causes heart disease amounts to *zero*. The same goes for the common myth that eating meat can cause cancer.

Even more impressive is to consider the fact that, for twenty years previously, Zoë had been a vegetarian. As a true scientist now faced with new facts, she abandoned that way of eating and became an advocate for an evidence-based, high-fat, low-carb diet.

If you have not heard of Zoë's groundbreaking work before, it should not come as a surprise, for reasons that should now be obvious.

On the other hand, advocates for eating more plants are given free airtime, even if they originate from a purely *ideological* position. One notable example is the Seventh-day Adventist Church (SDA).

The SDA was founded in 1863 after a teenage girl named Ellen G. White had a series of visions in which it was revealed to her that foods of animal origin were harmful morally, physically, and spiritually, and that only a diet based on plants was approved by God.

White authored a book *A Solemn Appeal to Mothers* that told America's moms that the best way to prevent the sin of masturbation was to abstain from eating meat, which she claimed was toxic and would stimulate immoral desires.

The typesetter of that book happened to be a young devotee of the church called John Harvey Kellogg, whose belief in the anti-masturbation properties of plant foods also drove him to create new foodstuffs from grains, as well as one of the earliest meat substitutes in 1896, "Nuttose", made from peanuts.

Kellogg would of course go on to build one of the world's largest ultra-processed food brands, which is very much in line with the SDA church's divinely-ordained mission. The SDA's followers believe that they have been charged by God to use business specifically as a tool to effect moral change in society. Ellen White herself also went on to found the Sanitarium corporation in Australia. Still owned by the SDA church, Sanitarium is the single biggest grain producer in Australasia.

Now it should be pointed out here that the SDA ideology is partly true! Eating a diet lacking in sufficient nutrition most certainly *does* curtail libido.

In fact, this would be proved by Ancel Keys' first foray into diet science, known as the Minnesota Starvation Experiment, which started around the same time he was commissioned to produce a ration pack for the US military. This experiment, which would probably be outlawed today, monitored a group of thirty-seven men as they lived on *half* their normal calorie intake over a twenty-four week period.

In addition to losing on average a quarter of their body weight, the results showed a general decrease in mental faculty, severe emotional stress and depression, along with significant loss of libido. Many of the participants would go on to suffer long-term negative effects for years after the experiment concluded.

Aside from curtailing sexual desire, a nutrient-poor diet also causes loss of basic physical and reproductive vitality, as evidenced by this report from tests run at California's Loma Linda University Medical Centre.

"We found that diet does significantly affect sperm quality. Vegetarian and vegan diets were associated with much lower sperm counts than omnivorous diets..." ~ Dr Eliza Orzylowska

The SDA's religiously-motivated philosophy that promotes a modern version of slave food continues to be a dominant force in the present day. In fact, the SDA church also owns or manages over a hundred fifty universities and colleges, making it the world's second largest educator after the Catholic Church.

Yet another area in which the SDA church continues covertly to exert significant influence over dietary education is through its ongoing involvement with various Dietetic Associations around the world.

The American Dietetic Association was founded in 1917 by Lenna Cooper and Lulu Graves. Cooper was a member of the SDA church, had been a follower of Kellogg's, and a strong advocate for vegetarianism. The ADA (which has since rebranded to the "Academy of Nutrition and Dietetics") continues to advocate for a wholly plant-based diet.

"It is the position of the American Dietetic Association that appropriately planned vegetarian diets, including total vegetarian or vegan diets, are healthful, nutritionally adequate, and may provide health benefits in the prevention and treatment of certain diseases."

For more evidence of how deep the influence of the anti-meat philosophy goes, we only have to look at the current members of the Dietary Guidelines Advisory committee, which is a group appointed every five years to update the science for the Dietary Guidelines for Americans. The most recent committee has five members, of which four have vested pro-plant or anti-meat interests: one describes herself as a "fan of plant-based meat alternatives"; another is professor of public health at Loma Linda University (which happens to be owned by the Seventh Day Adventist church); another is an active participant in a vegetarian advocacy group; and yet another previously sat on the advisory board of the agrochemical and agricultural biotechnology corporation Monsanto.

Despite having no scientific basis, the push to eat more plants now appears to be universal. *Everyone knows* we should have a "balanced diet". Every one of us has heard we should all be getting our "Five a day", however did you know this slogan has no basis in science but was in fact born out of a meeting of fruit and vegetable companies in California in 1991?

Let us move on to look at some of the health outcomes that proceed from following the national dietary guidelines.

The dietary guide   lines recommend that no more than 30% of energy intake should come from fats. As humans cannot source much energy from protein (15% maximum), that means *over half* of everyone's calorie needs must logically come from the only remaining macronutrient: carbohydrate.

Farmers have known for millennia that the quickest way to fatten up an animal, such as a steer, hog, or a goose, was to feed it an abundance of grains. For some reason, the same logic does not seem to apply to our species, yet just three crops: maize, wheat, and rice, now account for more than half of all the calories consumed by humans in the world today!

We are told to choose skim milk over whole milk, despite the fact that skim milk was, until recently, a by-product left over from the cream-making process that was fed to pigs, to help fatten them up for market, and of course despite the fact that whole milk has been shown to reduce heart attack risk.

When Zoë Harcombe analyzed forty of the most current studies looking at total fat and total saturated fat intake, the *only* statistically relevant finding was a positive correlation between the consumption of industrially-produced trans-fats and coronary heart disease.

Despite all the evidence, including a clear positive correlation between saturated fat and longevity in European countries, the campaign against fat carries on unabated. Even in 2010, US national recommendations continued to state that no more than seven percent of calorie intake should come from saturated fats.

Of course another thing *everyone knows* is that animal fat is pretty much synonymous with saturated fat, right? But what everybody *doesn't know* is that *every* source of fat found in nature combines all three types: saturated, monounsaturated, and polyunsaturated fats. What's more, there are only two sources that contain *more* saturates than unsaturates, which are milk and coconut oil.

The end result is that, today, a massive *two thirds* of what Americans eat qualifies as ultra-processed products, which are reconstituted primarily from nutrient-poor crops such as wheat, corn, seed oils, soy, and sugar.

In one year, the average American will now consume thirty-six pounds of oils (of which the vast majority are industrially-produced), one hundred forty-six pounds of flour, and—incredibly—even more sugar, a staggering one hundred fifty-two pounds each!

If two thirds of the U.S. diet is now factory-made feed, that means Americans must derive *practically all* their nutrition, including vitamins and crucial essential fatty acids, from just *one third* of their food. How is that possible?

Of all the significant modern changes in diet, one particular ingredient stands out from the rest: the seed oils.

At the beginning of the twentieth century, practically *all* America's dietary fat came from animal fat, with a little coconut oil. By 2005, eighty-six percent of added fats came from the new plant sources. And the trend continues: animal fat consumption is still dropping; plant-derived oil consumption is still going up. Today, about one in every three calories consumed in the United States now comes from this source, which had been practically unknown only a century ago, making it the most seismic shift in diet ever!

And yet we are supposed to believe that the present epidemic in chronic disease is a result of eating what humans have always eaten. In other words, ancestral foods now cause modern disease!

The reality is that the epidemic of obesity and chronic sickness has two primary dietary causes: nutrient deficiency and toxicity. Following the grain-based dietary guidelines will inevitably lead to nutrient deficiency, because you cannot meet one hundred percent of your nutritional needs from one third of your food.

As Weston A. Price's observations proved, the lack of nutrients, and fat-soluble vitamins in particular, inevitably leads to a rapid decline in the human condition. But the attack on human health also comes on a second front.

We are now consuming *highly toxic amounts* of omega-6 fats.

As previously mentioned, omega-6 fatty acids are essential in the diet, but only in small amounts, and in the correct proportions with the omega-3s.

Earlier we made reference to a paper published in the British Journal of Sports Medicine that showed that coronary heart disease is actually a chronic *inflammatory* condition. We know that omega-6 fats have inflammatory properties, which is why they must be balanced with appropriate amounts of the anti-inflammatory omega-3s.

That is exactly what our hunting ancestors will have gotten from nature. The fat of all wild, hoofed animals has an omega-6 component of two percent on average, up to a maximum of four percent. The net result is that omega-6s would have made up only about one percent of the ancestral diet.

The modern Western diet, as promoted by the national eating guidelines, will deliver between seven and twelve percent *linoleic acid alone!*

In those excess amounts, omega-6 fatty acids become *chronic toxins* to the body. Unlike *acute* toxins, which would produce an immediate reaction, a chronic toxin only starts to have an effect over time. The more omega-6 you consume, the more they build up in your body's tissues, leading to a significant imbalance and eventually to chronic inflammation.

We now know that atherosclerosis is also caused by *inflammation* in blood vessels that triggers the body's repair mechanisms, which use the much-maligned molecule cholesterol. That explains why John Gofman discovered cholesterol in damaged arteries back in the 1940s. The cholesterol did not *cause* the damage, any more than the presence of firefighters at a house fire means they started the blaze!

Considering that your liver actually synthesizes between 70 and 80% of the cholesterol your body needs raises one obvious question: why would your body create a chemical that clogged your arteries and could kill you?

The accumulation of omega-6 fats in the body also leads directly to obesity, as shown by a study published in the Journal of Nutrition in 1993. It gave the results of an experiment in which three groups of rats were fed almost identical diets over 3 weeks. The diets were the same in almost every respect, providing the same calorific, overall fat, and carbohydrate content. The only variable was the *type of fats* given.

• The rats that had been fed *beef tallow* (which contains 4.4% omega-6) ended the three weeks with 10.4% concentration of linoleic acid in their body fat.

• The group given *olive oil* (7.7% omega-6), gained 7.5% more body weight than the tallow group and finished with 15.2% linoleic acid in their body fat.

• The group given their fat in the form of *safflower oil* (which is 36.5% omega-6) finished with 54.5% linoleic acid concentration in their body fat. Furthermore, they gained an *additional* 12.3% in weight over the olive oil group, which is the equivalent to an average adult putting on twenty-one pounds in just three weeks!

This single experiment disproves the common, simplistic misconception that, at least in rats, fat gain is not a matter of "calories in versus calories out". There is no reason why the same should not be the case with humans.

In fact the same effect is now clearly observable in the human population. In 1959, the average linoleic acid content in the body fat of the U.S. population was 9.1%. By 2008, that figure had more than doubled to 21.5%, with the obesity rate also at 34%. (By 2015, only seven years later, we were already at almost forty percent obesity.)

If you look at the diets of today's remaining indigenous tribes that continue to consume their traditional foods, the total dietary linoleic acid content is never above two percent. As we have seen, in Westernized diets, that figure is between *seven and twelve percent.*

And that is not even the end of the dangers of excess omega-6. Macrophages are cells that specialize in removing damaged cells, including cancerous cells. Excess omega-6 fatty acids have been shown to inhibit the activity of macrophages to absorb the vitamin C they need to function properly. Now consider that, when the first seed oil food products were introduced at the turn of the last century, there was practically no cancer. Today we are told half of Americans can expect to get cancer in their lifetimes. Can that just be coincidence?

Type-2 diabetes has also exploded, increasing *twenty-five-fold* in the past eighty years. And coronary heart disease, practically unknown in the nineteenth century, is also now a major killer.

The net result is that today most of us are destined to be killed by some kind of chronic disease. In September 2011, the United Nations declared that, for the first time in human history, chronic non-communicable diseases such as heart disease, cancer, and diabetes pose a greater health burden worldwide than all infectious diseases, contributing to 35 million deaths annually.

There is also a growing body of scientists who are convinced that the prevalence of polyunsaturated omega-6 fatty acids in our diets is the single key cause of the majority of our health problems, even linking all chronic diseases to a common root cause.

Mitochondria are organelles that live inside all your cells and generate ninety percent of the energy your body needs via a complex called the *electron transport chain*. When too much omega-6 fatty acid accumulates in cells and mitochondria, this interrupts the electron transport chain and results in reduced cellular energy. That mitochondrial dysfunction has been implicated as a factor in *every* known chronic disease.

Is it any coincidence that there are only two categories of animal on Earth that suffer from obesity and chronic disease? They are human beings and our pets, the only other creatures that do not consume their natural, species-appropriate food.

Why?

Why have we stopped eating our species-appropriate diet? Why have we forgotten how to feed ourselves? Why have we allowed government to dictate it to us?

It's just business, economics, the basic law of supply and demand.

The huge surplus of cheap commodity ingredients meant the food System *had* to create corresponding demand. Advertising, official public guidelines, and even religion have been used to convince us that the fake, factory-made alternatives are somehow better than what nature provides.

We have all simply been *farmed*. In the eyes of the Owners, you and I are nothing more than consumers, and our sole purpose in life is to consume as much as possible.

Chapter 14:
Consumption Compulsion

Since the invention of agriculture, the System has always been dependent on constant expansion. It can only generate maximum profits for the Owners by consuming as many resources as possible as fast as possible.

When it comes to the diet that the centralized, intensified food education business tells us to eat, the prime objective is *consumption*. The food System wants each of us to consume more and more and more. Of course, as the System is inherently psychopathic, any impacts on human health and ecological health do not merit consideration. Only profits matter.

Make no mistake, all that matters to the System is that we obey the bullshit and eat what we are told to eat. That will continue to be good for profits even if it proves disastrous to our bodies and to our environment.

As far as the food System is concerned, our role is not as beneficiaries or stakeholders but as stock units, moving parts, and our sole purpose is consumption. Your purpose in life is to be a consumer, and the more you consume, the better.

It would even be a mistake to imagine that creating such dependency is an action exclusive to corporations. The interests and motivations of the corporations have long been inseparable from those of governments, and food is a major weapon of war. Consider, for example, that in 1873 the American government ordered the slaughter of 1.5 million buffalo for no other reason than to force the natives of the land to become more dependent on their new agricultural food System.

It is now obvious that the industrial feed we are eating and the rate at which we are consuming it is making the population chronically sick. But far from being a problem to the System, that is in fact another benefit, because the same Owners are happy to step in and sell us *additional products* that promise to counter the symptoms of the sickness. The sicker we get, the more insulin and statins and chemotherapy drugs they can sell. It really is the perfect win-win.

What the System does *not* want is for us to be able to meet our needs ourselves. It does not profit if we source healthy food from local producers, or when we take care of our own health. Its overall message is, "Don't worry about that stuff, we can sell you products to deal with that, pay here!"

"Don't worry about healthy food, that's expensive and time-consuming. We have far more convenient solutions. Pay here!"

"Don't worry about getting sick, we have pharmaceutical products to help manage the symptoms. Pay here!"

"And don't worry that half of you are going to get cancer. Together we can beat it, but only with your help to fund more research. Pay here!"

You really have to admire the brilliant way the System has proceeded to gain almost total control over our bodies, to the point where the majority will continue to trough on toxic fake food that can only make them sick without even noticing.

In this chapter, we will reveal how industrial fake food has been specifically and deliberately designed to keep you munching your way into chronic disease.

First, let's define what *real food* is. Real food gives your body the energy and the nourishment it requires. When your body has enough fuel and nutrition, it feels satiated, which means it does not need to keep eating, but instead can get on with other enjoyable activities.

That is desirable from your perspective, but it is undesirable from the point of view of the System, which thrives on endless consumption.

That's why modern, industrially produced, slave feed has been crafted *not* to nourish, satisfy, and satiate you, but the reverse. It is designed to make you continually crave more, and it achieves this in four simple ways.

1. Lack of Nutrition

The first element of the food addiction solution is what *is not* included: nutrition.

Being based on cheap, industrially-harvested commodity crops, human feed is inevitably devoid of nutrition: the minerals and vitamins, including the essential fat-soluble vitamins (A, D, and K) that are not present in any fats of plant origin.

We have already seen that today, two thirds of the Western diet is made up of ultra-processed, reconstituted commodity crops, which are naturally lacking in nutritional value, leading to an impossible equation where the remaining third of your plate must provide practically one hundred percent of the nutrients your body needs.

If the feed that you are given to eat is lacking in nutrients, leading inevitably to deficiencies, what is your body bound to do? It must keep telling you that it needs nourishment using the only communication tools it has: hunger and cravings.

So nutrient-deficient factory feed cannot and will not ever satisfy you, but you will continue to feel a constant biological urge to source the missing nutrients.

The second key factor works in much the same way.

2. Fake Salt

Everyone with a little science education knows that the chemical formula for salt is sodium chloride. But that is incorrect.

Sodium chloride is *a* salt: i.e. an electrically stable compound comprising a positively-charged ion (e.g. a metal such as sodium) joined to a negatively-charged ion (e.g. chloride).

Natural salt is a complex combination of many different salts, made up of a variety of metal and non-metal ions, many of which are vital to good health. Animals' instincts will drive them to travel many miles to find salt to lick, which can provide the spectrum of electrolytes they need. True salt is no less essential to human health, and in fact Roman soldiers were even paid in salt, giving us the word "salary".

If you pick up table salt from the grocery store, you are not getting that kind of natural salt, but just one *single* salt, which is not found in that form in nature but happens (yet again) to be an industrial byproduct.

A wide range of industrial processes depend on salts, including the creation of batteries, explosives, fertilizers, and plastics. For this reason, industrial plants were often located close to salt works. Various compounds (such as magnesium, potassium, calcium, bicarbonate, and iodide) would be extracted for a range of industrial applications and leaving behind copious quantities of the two most common ions present in seawater, which are, you guessed it, sodium and chloride.

Always looking for ways to reduce costs and increase profits, when the System has a surplus of something, it will look for a way to sell it. That's why we have fluoride in drinking water and toothpaste, not because it is good for health (it isn't, it is one of the most powerful toxins known to man), but because it was a problematic byproduct of the aluminum smelting industry that would have been very costly to dispose of safely.

That's why table salt on the shelves in your local store, as well as the "salt" component of practically all ultra-processed foods, is just sodium chloride. You don't get that pure chemical by evaporating seawater, or by mining the salts left behind by long-ago-dried-up oceans. You get it by taking those natural, full-spectrum salts and removing all the most profitable components.

Your body is almost certainly deficient in the numerous minerals that are lacking in the modern diet, many of which are salts, and that deficiency will lead to cravings. As we are still biologically Paleolithic, we will have the same response our ancestors did. When their bodies recognized a salt craving it drove them to seek out a natural source of salt, just like any other animal.

Today, our bodies are actually constantly crying out for the full range of salts and minerals they need, which drives us to consume foods with added salt. However what they are getting is not the natural combination they expect, complete with magnesium, potassium, iodine and the rest... just high quantities of one single salt. So again that means another craving that can never be satisfied.

Today's medical advice tells us we are all eating too much salt, but this is bullshit. We are actually *not consuming enough salt*! What we *are* getting is too much *sodium*!

Once again, it is all about imbalance. The dose makes the poison.

Your body is constantly trying to maintain a delicate balance between certain pairs of chemicals such as magnesium and calcium, and also sodium and potassium. Being chemically very similar, sodium and potassium compete with each other. An excess of sodium pushes potassium out of cells, interfering with the cells' normal ability to maintain water balance.

So the factory feed diet leaves us constantly craving vitamins, minerals, and salts, causing our bodies to cry out for the nutrition that is missing, but which can never be fulfilled, no matter how much ultra-processed food we consume.

But the design of this food is even more insidious, because it has been created specifically to be addictive, by playing tricks that take advantage of natural, ancestral, biological processes.

For many generations now, food scientists have known the secrets of making fake factory feed *hyper-palatable*.

3. Hyper-palatability

To understand how this works, let's look again at our natural, ancestral way of eating. For most of the year, our Paleolithic ancestors' diets would have consisted mainly of meat, organs, and animal fat. Because those types of foods are extremely nutrient-dense, that would leave them feeling satiated for long periods. So it would not be a problem to eat once per day, or maybe to feast on one day and then go without food for three.

However, at one particular time of year ("fat storage time") it makes evolutionary sense to consume as much extra energy as possible in order to store plenty of spare fat. In fact, the combination of available food at that time has particular properties that promote rapid fat storage.

In normal ancestral living, we would have typically eaten foods that contained *either* protein and fats together, *or* carbohydrates with a little protein, as there is actually no food that has zero protein component.

In fact, there are surprisingly few natural foods that combine *both* carbs and fats together! The only time you find this specific combination is in foods that nature *intends* to be consumed in quantity at certain specific times. The list is very short: only milk, nuts, seeds, and avocados.

Something about the combination of carbohydrates and fats together seems to bypass our natural satiation, thereby allowing a mammal to get as much nutrition and energy into her young as possible, or helping a plant to maximize its chances of broadcasting its genetics by having all its seeds or nuts eaten compulsively by animals.

Imagine if you were served plain, dry bread, you might eat a slice or two before it would get boring. The same is true with plain boiled rice or plain mashed potato. But if you add butter to the bread, fry the rice in oil, or mix butter and cream in with the potato, suddenly you would find you are able to eat far more in a sitting.

The modern food System had this formula figured out generations ago. So now, instead of being a rare, seasonal combination, the *majority* of processed fake foods now combine fats (predominantly in the form of cheap, industrial seed oils) with carbohydrates (from other cheap ingredients like refined sugars, flour, and corn syrup). The compulsive fat-carb combo is now our dietary *default*.

Think of all the foods that you just *know* are both fattening and easy to eat to excess: pancakes, waffles, cookies, cakes, chocolate, ice cream, pizza, hash browns, french fries, butter popcorn… every one of them combines fat with carbs.

The formula was figured out most notably by the researcher Howard Moskowitz, who described the exact proportions of sugar, salt, and fat to create what he coined the "bliss point", where natural satiation was bypassed, creating the ideal conditions for over-consumption.

Of course satiation is not good for profits. Processed feed products are not addictive by accident, it is quite deliberate. Anything that promotes compulsive and addictive consumption is better for the bottom line.

And one other recent refined product promotes addiction like no other: refined sugar!

4. Sweet Heroin

Both sugar and wheat are known to be addictive substances. Wheat contains an opioid that has been shown to affect the same part of the brain as heroin. Similarly, any time sugar is consumed, the reward hormone dopamine is released in the brain, giving a short-term high. However repeated use actually suppresses dopamine signaling, which decreases the pleasure signals the brain receives, leading over time to more compulsive behavior.

Sugar also makes it harder for the brain to suppress the hunger-signaling hormone ghrelin and interferes with the normal function of another hormone, leptin, which is the one that helps to produce the feeling of satiety.

Ancestrally, sugar would have been a rare treat, found on its own, in the form of honey, or in fruit (combined with extra vitamin C). It should also be noted that nature never combines sugar with significant amounts of either starch or protein.

Mammals do receive sugar combined with fat, for a limited period, through their mother's milk. Milk is high in the sugar lactose, which helps, along with the high concentration of saturated fats, to promote rapid brain development.

Sugar was never naturally meant to be consumed over an extended period. Consuming any amount causes a "sugar high", followed by a necessary release of insulin to lower the blood sugar levels, which leads to an energy crash, and that in turn drives cravings for more sugar.

Frequent consumption of refined sugar also alters the balance of bacteria in the gut, to the detriment of certain bacteria that manufacture the B vitamins that are essential to proper brain function, inevitably leading to diminished mental and memory performance.

Some scientists, including Doctors Abram Hoffer, Allan Cott, and Linus Pauling, have even claimed that *all* mental disorders can be directly linked to the effects of sugar dependency. It may be no coincidence that the first mental asylums were only introduced in Britain at the end of the seventeenth century, following a period of rapid expansion in the availability of mass-produced, refined sugar.

Other researchers, including Dr. Thomas Seyfried Ph.D, have made the link between sugar and the growth of cancers, specifically exploring how the vast majority of cancer cells only have the ability to metabolize either glucose (from sugar), while a few can also use the amino acid glutamine.

Sugar has also been indicted in the recent explosion in non-alcoholic fatty liver disease and other chronic disorders. Sucrose, table sugar, comprises one glucose and one fructose molecule. While every living cell has the ability to metabolize glucose, your cells cannot use fructose. The only way your body can deal with fructose is to convert it to glycogen and also fats, some of which are stored in the liver, which can lead to non-alcoholic fatty liver disease.

A healthy person will only ever have a total of four grams—approximately a *single teaspoon*—of glucose in their entire bloodstream.

If there is any more present, it is the liver's job to remove the excess, which it can store as glycogen for later release. But prolonged high intake of refined sugar causes the liver rapidly to reach capacity and so any surplus sugar is converted into fatty acids that are stored in the least active parts of the body (belly, buttocks, thighs, and breasts), and also around the organs as visceral fat, excess amounts of which are harmful to health.

Despite the growing evidence of negative health impacts, due to its uniquely appealing qualities, the prevalence of sugar in the Western diet has continued to accelerate in recent years, to the point where it is now present in *almost everything.*

Dr. Robert Lustig of the University of California estimates that an incredible *eighty percent* of the 600,000 food products offered for sale on U.S. shelves today now contain *added sugar*! People in many parts of the world are now consuming an average of more than 500 calories per day from *added* sugar alone.

We have seen that the ingredients preferred by the industrial feed system for their cheapness and convenience also result in a plethora of new grocery items that fundamentally lack nutrition, are therefore unable truly to satisfy our hunger, plus are combined and packaged in a way that promotes compulsive, addictive consumption.

Modern fake foods are a *facsimile* of food. They are designed to manipulate our natural biological desires for nutrition, flavor, and texture, yet without ever fulfilling our real needs.

The fact that every feature of these products is *by design* is how we define "ultra-processed foods". Of course humans have processed our food for countless millennia, primarily to get it to last longer and go further. The majority of our culinary processes have their origins in the need for preservation including drying, smoking, salting or brining, pickling, and fermenting.

Ultra-processed foods go far beyond these basic preservation processes, which still retain the essential characteristics of the original foodstuff. Ultra-processed products are designed to mimic real food. Their flavor profiles, appearance, and texture are not inherent to any natural food, but are rather the product of industrial design, and often with an eye to hyper-palatability.

"The problem is we are not eating food anymore, we are eating food-like products." ~ Dr. Alejandro Junger

This is, of course, all good for the profits of the food System and the Owners.

Fake feed is simply more profitable than nature's food. The enormous profits it generates allow the creation of food brands, ultimately owned by a relatively small number of massive corporations, that can afford to invest the huge sums required to dominate the mass market.

The effective monopolies these same corporations enjoy also mean they can dictate not just the dietary guidelines but also the messages that come over the airwaves with catchy advertising slogans and jingles. And the public continues to lap it up. Even though they tell us that once we pop, we can't stop, we continue to drop those tubes of God-knows-what into our trolleys.

We have even let the System get its claws into our babies, forgoing the food nature gave us, which worked perfectly for millions of years, in favor of the convenience of lab-produced "formula", a name that does not even attempt to hide the fact that it is a completely artificial facsimile of the real thing.

It is not even as though there is any lack of evidence of the catastrophic effects of the modern diet. There are plenty of documentaries and first-hand accounts out there from people who have switched to an all-ultra-processed diet for a few weeks, with consistently shocking results. Of course, these outlier reports will never make the mainstream, you will have to go digging to find them, and the System will always ensure they are drowned out by the official narrative that shouts from every billboard how meat will kill you, how you must limit saturated fat and instead ensure you get your "heart-healthy" grains and polyunsaturated fats.

Still, when almost half of us are now obese, we are told it must be our fault, that we have failed to count our calories, and that we need to "go on a diet". The modern bullshit concept of "dieting" actually fails more than ninety percent of the time, leading to yo-yoing weight loss followed by rebounding weight gain (which has also been shown to damage health and shorten lifespan), with dieters coming out the other side miserable, disillusioned, guilt-wracked, and even more nutrient-depleted.

Now that two thirds of what we eat is ultra-processed, is it possible that we have forgotten what food is even supposed to taste like? Most of us have certainly lost the ability to recognize real food, how to prepare it with time, love, and care in our own kitchens, and the value of sitting down every evening to share good, honest, real food with our families and loved ones.

Yet we can take comfort in knowing we are each playing our vital part in supporting the System, as consumers, or in the words of Dr. Henry Kissinger, "useless eaters".

No poet has summed up the Western addiction to consumption more elegantly than the late, great George Carlin.

"America the beautiful: one big, transcontinental commercial cesspool. And how do the people feel about all this? How do the people feel about living in a coast-to-coast shopping mall?

Well they think it's all **JUST FUCKIN' DANDY**!

They think it is cool as can be, because Americans love the mall, they love the mall. That's where they get to satisfy their two most prominent addictions at the same time: shopping and eating.

Millions of semi-conscious Americans day after day shuffling through the malls shopping and eating, especially eating. Americans love to eat. They are fatally attracted to the slow death of fast food...

These people are efficient, professional, compulsive consumers. That's their civic duty: consumption…

The only true, lasting American value that's left, buying things! People spending money they don't have on things they don't need."

And so many of us are proud to play our part in supporting "the economy". We toe the line, secure in the knowledge that our leaders are there to protect and to serve *us*, that it is their priority to look after our freedoms and our wellbeing.

We are happy to step up and pay the price, first with our post-tax earnings, and then yet again with our health.

What will it take for the people to wake up to the fact that the artificial feed we have been told to eat for the past few generations is robbing us of our life and vitality and slowly killing us?

What needs to happen to break the spell that the government truly does not, and in fact *cannot*, care about our health, wellbeing, and happiness?

To try and answer these questions, we are now going to take a peek behind the curtain and contemplate one possible logical answer... What if there really *is* no government? What if all that is left are corporations?

Chapter 15:
Useless Eaters

At this point you may feel like you are standing at a crossroads, experiencing what psychologists call "cognitive dissonance". On one hand, you have been told your whole life that society is set up to work for your best interests, for your freedom, health, wealth, and opportunity. Yet so much evidence now seems to point the other way.

In this chapter we will show why it just does not add up, why our society surely does not, and cannot, work in the ultimate interests of the people.

There are simply too many contradictions, too many inconsistencies, but these all begin to make sense once you realize that the corporations have completely taken over.

As soon as you *really* accept that fact, and that furthermore there is no cavalry coming to your aid, you will have taken a crucial step towards freedom, and you will be in a position to make better choices for yourself and your family.

The only reason the population has not come to the realization that practically everything is now owned and controlled by massive corporations is because we are surrounded by wall-to-wall, 24/7 bullshit, traditionally known as propaganda.

The following quote is from the pen of Edward Bernays, but could easily have been written by Machiavelli centuries earlier.

"Intelligent men must realize that propaganda is the modern instrument by which they can fight for productive ends and help to bring order out of chaos."

It has always been far easier to control the people through manipulation of the narrative than by force. Machiavelli knew it; Joseph Goebbels knew it; Stalin knew it; Edward Bernays knew it… Propaganda is the System's primary tool of domination.

How do we hear what is going on in the world today? How do we make up our minds about what to believe? It comes almost exclusively from the government, non-governmental organizations, and the media, all of which are entirely corporate-controlled.

The whole political pantomime exists to give the impression that all levels of government are busy working to make things better. But despite all the theater of party politics, all the arguing and tinkering with small matters, all the time in the background the real business of the day, the Owners' final power grab, is nearing completion.

Governments used to keep corporations in check by limiting their charters and prohibiting monopolies. Is it possible that the tables have turned and that corporations now run government?

That idea becomes more credible when you realize government is run by human beings, and individuals who are drawn to politics are too often ambitious, selfish, and easily corrupted. Once a corporation has enough resources, and there is enough profit at stake, it is a simple matter to bribe a politician to push the corporate agenda with promises of campaign funding or lucrative private sector directorships.

Today, the corporations have more than enough resources, so any costs to the business, compared to the individual's perceived gain and therefore the potential leverage the money can exert, are trivial. Buying political influence is a simple, convenient, legal, and highly profitable investment.

Most people believe we can trust non-profit organizations to look after our interests. Like the American Heart Association, for example? But remember that body only gained its national influence thanks to massive sponsorship from Procter & Gamble, the manufacturer of trans-fat-laden Crisco, which managed to get away with selling its toxic product for ninety-five years before it was replaced. Or maybe the American Dietetic Association, which we know has been controlled by the SDA church since its inception?

Corporations are in the business of buying influence to further their agendas. It is simply an extremely cost-effective form of PR and marketing.

What about the independent regulators that exist to protect individual consumers from abuse by large corporations? In fact the reverse is the rule: regulation too often protects the interests of the larger corporations *from* the people.

146

Let's go back to the food sector and take the example of raw milk. People had been perfectly healthy consuming raw dairy for thousands of years until 1924 when new regulations came in that purported to protect the nation's health by requiring milk to be pasteurized, effectively outlawing the sale of raw dairy products (which is still the case in much of the US). The new requirement made it impractical for small dairy farmers, who could not afford their own pasteurization facilities, to continue to do business, pushing them out of the market in favor of large-scale industrial producers.

One of the easiest ways to verify the utter lack of credibility in the arena of regulation is to look at the foot traffic between any large industry and its respective governmental regulatory body. As the Open Secrets website explains:

"Although the influence powerhouses that line Washington's K Street are just a few miles from the US Capitol building, the most direct path between the two doesn't necessarily involve public transportation. Instead, it's through a door—a revolving door that shuffles former federal employees into jobs as lobbyists, consultants and strategists just as the door pulls former hired guns into government careers."

Spend a little time browsing the Open Secrets website and you will soon realize that, not only is this practice commonplace, but that no attempt is made to hide it, because it is entirely legal.

Don't we have protections above the national level? What about all the non-governmental organizations (NGOs) that appear to wield even more power than individual governments? Consider bodies such as the United Nations, the World Bank, or the World Health Organization. Who elects them? To whom are they ultimately accountable? If you cannot answer those questions, you should assume it isn't you.

In the words of George Carlin, "It's a big club... and you're not in it!"

Consider that the second biggest backer of the World Health Organization is the Bill and Melinda Gates Foundation. Does it not seem absurd that a business oligarch should be able effectively to buy potential influence over a non-governmental organization that itself wields enough power to direct the actions of entire governments across the globe?

At least we have a free press to keep us informed. In the modern world we have always been able to turn to the media to give us the facts. However, our press, which may once have enjoyed freedom, is also now almost entirely corporate-owned. In fact the majority of global media brands belong to just *six* massive corporations. Between them, Comcast, Disney, TimeWarner, NewsCorp, National Amusements, and Sony have a combined worth of $430 billion and own practically every news and entertainment brand you can think of.

Not even state-owned broadcasters can be viewed as independent. On September 11, 2001, the British BBC announced that the Solomon Building, also known as WTC7, had collapsed, twenty-six minutes *before* it came down. Whatever explanation may be offered, two simple, chilling facts remain: first, some third party knew what was going to happen ahead of time; and then was also in a position to dictate what the "news" was going to be to a state broadcaster.

That is no conspiracy theory, it is evidence of a conspiracy. And the Owners will even speak openly about the immense value their control of the media confers.

"We are grateful to the Washington Post, the New York Times, Time Magazine and other great publications whose directors have attended our meetings and respected their promises of discretion for almost 40 years... It would have been impossible for us to develop our plan for the world if we had been subjected to the lights of publicity during those years. But, the world is more sophisticated and prepared to march towards a world government. The supernational sovereignty of an intellectual elite and world bankers is surely preferable to the national autodetermination practiced in past centuries." ~ David Rockefeller, speaking at a meeting of the Bilderberg Group in June, 1991

What about the Internet and social media, where we can be free to do our own research and to share ideas in a huge spectrum of interest groups? In reality, the major platforms are owned by some of the world's most massive corporations, who then have immense power to control which messages get seen and which get hidden. Then there's the army of so-called "fact checkers", today's equivalent to the "thought police" George Orwell described in Nineteen-Eighty Four, whose job it is to control the speech, actions, and thought of the population, defining unapproved thoughts as "thoughtcrime" (in today's parlance, "fake news").

But surely we can always rely on science to give us the straight facts! Interestingly, the idea that it is the job of science to give us conclusions and to tell us what to think misses the whole point of science.

Science is a process of learning more, but what you discover depends on the original motives and what you set out to find. Everyone employs scientists, from junk food and cosmetics manufacturers to fracking companies to Hitler's Third Reich... The fact that a scientist is involved in the endeavor does not automatically make the endeavor worthwhile or credible.

Because it is not a destination but a journey of constant inquiry, science can also never be truly "settled". There is always more to learn. In the words of a true scientist, Richard Feynman, one of the pioneers of quantum mechanics:

"I would rather have questions that can't be answered than answers that can't be questioned."

Compare this quote from a corporate-sponsored career scientist, Dr. Anthony Fauci, who here invokes *scientism*, the idea that science is some unimpeachable, religious authority that may not be questioned!

"A lot of what you're seeing as attacks on me quite frankly are attacks on science."

As we have seen, there is some real science going on, but the vast majority of research unfortunately is still dependent on corporate sponsorship. Universities rely to a large extent on corporate funding, and that investment is invariably tied to set outcomes, which demand the search for specific conclusions that support the sponsor's commercial objectives, leading one academic we interviewed to comment, "I don't know anywhere that real scientific research is going on in this country today."

We have seen time and time again that, even if they do get published, scientific findings that go against the corporate narrative are suppressed in favor of those that support the narrative, even ones that have been conclusively and consistently disproved.

We must accept the fact that we now find ourselves at a point where the Owners' incredible wealth has taken over *every single mainstream channel*.

As George Carlin explained...

"They own everything. They own all the important land. They own and control the corporations. They've long since bought and paid for the senate, the congress, the state houses, the city halls, they've got the judges in their back pockets and they own all the big media companies so they control just about all of the news and information you get to hear. They've got you by the balls! They spend billions of dollars every year lobbying, lobbying to get what they want. Well, we know what they want. They want more for themselves and less for everybody else."

But how did we get here? How did corporations become so big and powerful? It did not happen overnight, but gradually over the past couple hundred years.

Step back and look at history and you will see a clear trend. Over time, power has progressively become more centralized and, at the same time, more remote and untouchable.

It started with the original invention of legal corporations that abstracted the power of kings and queens away from specific individuals to inaccessible boards and shareholders and hedge funds. Now, even if the people wanted to revolt, there is no palace to storm.

Whereas states had always previously retained the power to limit or to dissolve a corporation, at the end of the 19th century corporations effectively achieved immortality when in 1896 the state of New Jersey passed a statute allowing corporations independently to define the *scope of their own charters*.

Now free from the shackles of limited charters, and following the Pareto principle, larger businesses could proceed to push out smaller competitors and gain increasing market share, which inevitably led to monopolies, such as John D. Rockefeller's Standard Oil, Andrew Carnegie's U.S. Steel, and Union Pacific under Edward H. Harriman.

After the U.S. government was forced to intervene to break up monopolies, in the interests of both the customer and the market, the industrialists found new ways to maintain their influence. They channeled some of their immense wealth into so-called charitable foundations, which could then invest in philanthropic endeavors apparently for the benefit of the general population.

One of the areas in which the Rockefeller Foundation bought influence was in medical education, using charitable bequests to buy seats on the board of every medical school. That indirect, but very real, financial influence could then be leveraged to promote an allopathic medical education system that focused exclusively on the new industry of pharmaceuticals, one in which Rockefeller happened to be heavily invested.

Another entrepreneur would apply the exact same strategy a century later. When the Microsoft Corporation was also hit by a massive antitrust suit, Bill Gates poured his wealth into the Bill and Melinda Gates Foundation, which promotes, among many other things, global vaccination programs. Gates also happens to be a major investor in pharmaceutical companies that manufacture vaccines. Oh, and of course we mentioned he *also* happens to be the second biggest funder of the WHO.

Perhaps he does all this to further the Gates Foundation's stated vision that every living being is equal. Or maybe it is just good business. Nevertheless, the freedom to move funds through foundations and other organizations is just one legal trick that effectively removes the barriers to how much influence individuals can exert over the market, and all highly tax-efficiently of course.

Corporations gained even more freedom to use their profits to influence public opinion, gaining the right to free speech *as individuals under law*, when in the 2010 case *Citizens United v. FEC*, the Supreme Court held that corporations have a political right to free speech under the First Amendment, including the right to "use money amassed from the economic marketplace to fund their speech".

We must conclude that, today, government is no longer by the people for the people, but rather *by the corporations for the corporations*.

Nothing sums up the current situation better than this speech, which comes from the 1976 movie *Network*, where capitalist business owner Ned Beatty explains to Howard Beale how the world really works.

"You are an old man who thinks in terms of nations and peoples. There are no nations! There are no peoples! There are no Russians. There are no Arabs. There are no third worlds. There is no West!

There is only one holistic system of systems, one vast and immane, interwoven, interacting, multivariate, multinational dominion of dollars. Petro-dollars, electro-dollars, multi-dollars, reichsmarks, rins, rubles, pounds, and shekels. It is the international system of currency which determines the totality of life on this planet. That is the natural order of things today...

There is no America. There is no democracy. There is only IBM and ITT and AT&T and DuPont, Dow, Union Carbide, and Exxon. Those are the nations of the world today...

The world is a college of corporations, inexorably determined by the immutable bylaws of business. The world is a business, Mr. Beale. It has been since man crawled out of the slime... One vast and ecumenical holding company, for whom all men will work to serve a common profit."

Once the final limits to corporate growth had been removed, there could be only one outcome. If you compare the GDP of nations alongside the annual revenues of big business, half of the world's largest economies are now private corporations. As Ned Beatty proclaimed almost fifty years ago, "Those are the nations of the world today."

Ultimately, though, all this is theory and history, and of course you cannot implicitly trust anything you read. Is there any way really to *know* whether society is working for us... or against us?

Yes. You only have to put aside what the System *says*, and instead just step back and look at what it *does*, to realize that, for all the noise and chatter, it only pays lip service to the stuff that really matters.

For example, we have already heard from David Montgomery that there is plenty of evidence showing that soil destruction seems to have been the single biggest cause of the demise of every previous great civilization. How much do you hear about the very real threat to humanity caused by soil loss from industrial agriculture? Next to nothing! What are we told? That farting cows are killing the planet!

152

What about the very real epidemics of obesity, coronary heart disease, diabetes, and cancer that are set to end the lives of more than half of us, despite being practically unknown just a century ago? They are raised as "major concerns", of course, but where are the proposed solutions? All we are told is that more research is clearly needed... but in the meantime, here, take these pills to lower your cholesterol!

Everything, from paleontology to simple common sense, points to our recent switch over to industrial "frankenfood" as the single most significant factor in our catastrophic collapse in health. Yet... crickets. Why?

The simple answer is that everything you have been told about food comes from corporations: the corporate-sponsored NGOs, regulators, dietary guidelines, scientists... And you *know* that corporations legally *cannot* put your health first, if it could harm profits.

That's why all the mainstream channels are *prohibited* from telling us simply to eat our ancestral diet, but instead must keep repeating the unfounded false dogmas that fat causes heart disease and meat causes cancer.

In 2015 we all heard about the International Agency for Research on Cancer's conclusion that red meat is "probably carcinogenic", yet what we were not told was that that claim was never, and has since never been, substantiated. The headlines proclaimed a terrifying "14% increased risk of cancer" if you consumed meat. But the actual results were so fundamentally weak they never merited a single column inch.

Aside from being based on an epidemiological study, which compared groups by their personal reports on lifestyle, and thereby one of the least reliable tests, the limited evidence pointed only to a positive *association* (which is absolutely not evidence of causation), and that the increased risk was only *relative risk*, a 14% variation from an already very small original risk, therefore a negligible difference. In these kinds of studies, only an increase in relative risk of *at least one hundred percent* would even merit further investigation into potential causation. Anything less is statistically insignificant, background noise.

Yet... headlines all around the world loudly proclaimed red meat to be "a probable carcinogen".

This is proof positive that the corporate-owned System is determined to sell you nothing but bullshit.

But surely there is a last port of call for truly independent health advice. Of course you can always trust the family doctor!

Yes, we are told that, but the truth is doctors get practically no training in nutrition, or in any area of preventative healthcare at all! Remember how Rockefeller used his foundation to take over medical education? Since then, all licensed doctors have received their training from a medical education system that for the past century has been owned by the Rockefeller-Carnegie pharma cartel. Because that system is only concerned with how to treat the symptoms of disease with drugs, that is all doctors are taught.

If a doctor wants to follow science and discover truths for themselves, even then the corporate-run System will intervene!

Dr Gary Fettke is an orthopedic surgeon who practices in Tasmania, Australia. After suffering pituitary cancer and undergoing chemotherapy for eleven years, Gary discovered the benefits of a low-carbohydrate diet and was able to put his own cancer into remission.

As he saw many of his own patients suffering from metabolic disease and diabetes, all too often resulting in amputations, Gary went on to explore the effectiveness of cutting out dietary carbohydrates in his patients, and was starting to see encouraging results.

But then came the bombshell. Gary received notice from the Tasmanian Medical Board informing him he was *legally prohibited* from giving his patients advice on nutrition! No evidence of harm was ever presented, so what was the motive for this intervention?

The ban would later be overturned by the High Court, but only after more than four years of battles. This experience prompted Gary's wife Belinda to delve into the world of dietary research and to become another outlier educator worth following. (If you look up Belinda's talks you can hear her explain how practically *all* dietary research today is sponsored by corporate vested interests.)

The System has proved by its deeds that it has interest in tackling the chronic disease epidemic. Of course it has to *pretend* to try, but the reality is it cannot interfere, not if that would put profits at risk.

That is why over the years scientists and doctors have been paid to tell us that smoking is healthy, that it's fat not sugar that causes coronary heart disease, or that weed killers that cause cancer are perfectly safe. Is there any reason to believe those practices are not continuing to the present day?

The bottom line is that it is far more profitable to make cheap products that destroy health and then to use bullshit to drive demand than it is to make healthy products in the first place. That's because there simply is not much profit in nature, and in nature's model health was always free.

The final nail in this coffin should be the UK's 1939 Cancer Act, which, under the guise of protecting the public, made it a criminal offense for anyone except a licensed physician to claim that *any* treatment can be effective against cancer. The System has even made curing a killer disease a crime.

This makes more sense when you appreciate the scale of the healthcare sector, and of course how industrial food and chronic health conditions are inextricably linked.

The international food trade is worth two trillion dollars a year, according to the UN's FAO. But there is also a lot of money to be made in *sickness*. Plus many of the Owners are heavily invested in both the health industry and food industry. (To understand more about how the same interests have fingers in all the pies, we recommend you look into the mind-boggling investment portfolios of certain funds, starting with Blackrock and Vanguard.)

How big is the pharma sector worldwide? You may be shocked to know it isn't far behind food, generating 1.27 trillion dollars in 2020 according to some estimates.

In 2019, one single drug, Lipitor, which lowers cholesterol, generated nearly two billion U.S. dollars of revenue for its owner Pfizer. That is, of course, despite the fact that we now know that higher cholesterol levels are associated with *longer life expectancy* in older people. But don't expect to hear that from your family doctor.

We now live on Planet Earth Incorporated. The corporations do not only provide the vast majority of what is sold as food, but they even control the flow of information, so what you are told to eat is corporate propaganda. And, once you get sick, they are waiting to sell you insulin and beta blockers and statins, so the System profits *twice*.

Many of today's corporations are bigger than governments and they now operate on a truly global scale. Everything, from money to energy to raw materials to the food supply, is now at once globalized and more centralized. Governments are now inconsequential players, the executive arms of the trans-national corporations and NGOs.

The Owners' personal fortunes have followed suit. Wealth inequality started to skyrocket in the 1970s, and has now stretched to astronomical proportions. According to a report published by Oxfam in 2017, "Eight men own the same wealth as the 3.6 billion people who make up the poorest half of humanity."

In 1971, a university professor named Klaus Schwab wrote a book with the uninspiring title *Moderne Unternehmensführung im Maschinenbau ("Modern Enterprise Management in Mechanical Engineering")*.

"In that book, he argued that the management of a modern enterprise must serve not only shareholders but all stakeholders (die Interessenten), to achieve long-term growth and prosperity."

In the very same year, Schwab also founded a group known as the World Economic Forum, whose members represent major governments and all the biggest multinational corporations. The World Economic Forum meets once a year in Davos, Switzerland to discuss global affairs and policy.

"Schwab has championed the multistakeholder concept since the Forum's inception, and it has become the world's foremost platform for public and private cooperation."

With its motto "Committed to improving the state of the world" the WEF's idea is that corporations must now be responsible to all their customers, suppliers, employees, and local communities. This all sounds positive, but it raises some tricky questions.

After enjoying deregulation and expanding to become bigger and more powerful than entire countries, are we to assume that the world's major corporations all collectively developed a sense

156

of social conscience and jumped merrily on board the responsibility bandwagon?

Also, who is Klaus Schwab, and how did a previously little-known academic suddenly come to be the leading figure in such a powerful global organization? The answer may lie in the roots of his early education.

According to his Wikipedia entry, while studying at Harvard, Schwab began what he described as a 50-year mentorship under a certain Dr. Henry Kissinger. Kissinger, who served as Secretary of State under Nixon, describes himself as being proud to be the "architect of the New World Order", and was also quoted as saying, "Who controls the food supply controls the people."

You get some insight into Kissinger's views on the average member of the public from the fact that, in his book *The Final Days*, which he has said may not be published until five years after his death, he reportedly refers to the elderly as "useless eaters".

Henry Kissinger was the author of the National Security Study Memorandum #200, popularly known as "The Kissinger Report", which was only made public when it was declassified and was transferred to the U.S. National Archives in 1990.

A collaboration between the CIA, the United States Agency for International Development (USAID), and the Departments of State, Defense, and Agriculture, the subject of the report was "Implications of Worldwide Population Growth for U.S. Security and Overseas Interests". It too implies that there are too many of these "useless eaters" consuming valuable resources that would be better used by a *reduced world population*.

In 2010 Kissinger's protégé Schwab authored a report for the WEF that argued that governments were no longer the dominant actors on the world stage and declared the time had come for a new stakeholder paradigm of international governance for a globalized world. This new order would be managed most effectively by a coalition of multinational corporations and governments through the United Nations and a few select "civil society organizations".

In 2020, the World Economic Forum met in Davos and announced "The Great Reset", which made a number of predictions about what would come to pass in the following decade, including the disquieting headline, "You will own nothing, and you will be happy."

This Great Reset is a revolution that, according to Schwab, "will come at a breathtaking speed, like a tsunami."

But what will this proposed future look like for the normal man and woman? What will it mean to own nothing?

The answer is not hidden. In fact it has been staring us in the face for years, in global macro-economics.

Our current financial system dates back just over a century to 1913 when the Fabian Society drew up the Federal Reserve Act, effectively handing the US economy over to a cartel of international financiers.

Previously, money had always represented real assets like gold and silver. As it takes a lot of labor to mine precious metals out of the ground, that conferred on money an intrinsic real-world benchmark value. You could work for a dollar, or alternatively you could choose to try to pan for a dollar's worth of gold. The money represented the gold, which in turn represented a real, measurable amount of work.

Just prior to World War One, the Owners introduced a totally different *unbacked* system that was based only on debt. Under the new system, currency only had value because somebody said it did, hence the name "fiat currency" ("fiat" is Latin for "let it be").

Under the fiat system, central banks like the newly formed Federal Reserve could print as much currency into existence as they wished, which they would then lend as a loan with interest to governments, corporations and individuals via the banking system.

But that created a problem. If all the dollars in the system originated from the Fed (a private corporation), how could the borrowed money—plus interest—ever get repaid? Of course that would be impossible, as the repayment would amount to more than all the money in existence! Therefore any economy based on this fiat currency is fundamentally bankrupt from day one.

So, to maintain the illusion, the central banks had to keep pumping exponentially more money into the system, always increasing the nation's debt. This of course created inflation, which is why a dollar in your hand today is worth only about one percent of a dollar in 1913, in real terms.

Eventually, the financial system would inevitably have to collapse. Considering that major Western economies have created more new currency just in the past two years since the start of the COVID crisis than every year in the previous century combined, it is not unreasonable to imagine that the collapse will be imminent.

Taking all the evidence into account... the System's unwillingness to tackle the health crisis; the unconscionable wealth inequality; the announcement of a Great Reset bringing in a New World Order; and the inevitable economic time bomb... we surely find ourselves at a unique point in history, facing the final days of the last great empire.

The process is now complete. The System has taken everything it can take.

At least we now have an answer to the big question, which is, if the System is so clearly unsustainable on every level from the soil to human health, why "they" didn't notice and do something. The answer is, they know, but the System was never set up to go on forever.

The Owners may be many things, but dumb is not one of them. Of course they knew it was never sustainable, and their response has been to double down on the power grab, leading up to this Great Reset, hidden behind the bullshit smokescreen of stakeholder inclusion, all the time secure in the knowledge that they have a final end game.

What should concern each of us right now is the role that has been ordained for us individually in the Owners' vision of the future. Now we no longer even hold the status of "consumers"; from the System's perspective we are nothing more than "useless eaters", and it appears we are surplus to requirements.

Chapter 16:
The War on Meat

"The world is ready for a world government. The supranational sovereignty of an intellectual elite and world bankers is certainly preferable to the national self-determination practiced in past centuries… We are on the verge of a global transformation. All we need is the 'right' global crisis and the nations will accept the New World Order." ~ David Rockefeller

The System's consolidation is practically complete. We are witnessing the end of a transition process away from multiple nations into a single, global empire, one built on a model that was always destined eventually to implode.

The question each of us must now ask is, what kind of future do they have in store for *us*? In this chapter, we will look at the available facts so that you can picture the various future paths available to humanity, and more importantly to you and your family, and then be in a position to make better-informed choices.

The first worrying signal we must consider concerns the possible size of the human population under the New World Order. There is actually a significant amount of evidence that the Owners are planning for, or would at the very least prefer, a massive reduction in our numbers.

Let's put human population density into historical context. In ancestral times, we could not afford to overpopulate as that would create the risk of overhunting our food sources. Once the weather warmed up and we switched to agriculture, creating an apparent abundance of calories, human labor became the limiting factor to growth so it made sense to breed much faster.

While the Industrial Revolution and the mechanization of agriculture facilitated a huge explosion in population, they also tipped the balance back the other way. Because machines enabled us to mine the earth's assets faster and more efficiently than ever, that required fewer bodies. Still, the majority would continue to play a useful role, dutifully consuming the industrial feed and paying their taxes, until such a point as wealth inequality would reach a tipping point with the Owners left holding all the real assets, such as Bill Gates who recently became the single biggest owner of US farmland with 242,000 acres.

At that point, they would not need the majority of us anymore! At that point, a large and impoverished human population of eight billion would surely constitute more of a threat than an asset.

This is more than mere speculation, we have it in their own words. Here is just a handful of examples from recent years.

"First we got population. The world today has 6.8 billion people. That's headed up to about 9 billion. Now if we do a really great job on new vaccines, health care, reproductive health services, we lower that by perhaps ten or fifteen percent." ~ Bill Gates, in his TED talk "Innovating to Zero" 2010

"A total world population of 250-300 million people, a 95% decline from present levels, would be ideal." ~ Ted Turner, founder of CNN

"The Planetary Regime might be given responsibility for determining the optimum population for the world and for each region and for arbitrating various countries' shares within their regional limits. Control of population size might remain the responsibility of each government, but the Regime would have some power to enforce the agreed limits." ~ From the book *Ecoscience*, co-authored by President Obama's Science czar, John P. Holdren

"Maintain humanity under 500,000,000 in perpetual balance with nature." ~ The Georgia Guidestones (erected anonymously in 1980 and also demolished anonymously in 2022)

The individuals who provided those quotes represent a System that has replaced the public's traditional food with factory-made fake alternatives, leading to a sudden and catastrophic decline in health. And here they are openly talking about the necessity of reducing our numbers. We truly are "useless eaters" to them.

Is it conceivable to continue to hold on to the belief that they can possibly care about your life, or the lives of your children and their children? No, instead the media ironically has us arguing among ourselves about whose lives matter!

"And even when they became discontented, as they sometimes did, their discontent led nowhere, because being without general ideas, they could only focus it on petty specific grievances. The larger evils invariably escaped their notice." ~ George Orwell, Nineteen Eighty Four

To be fair, we must admit the Owners are not entirely wrong in their "useless eaters" point of view. There are always truths in between the layers of bullshit, that is how bullshit works. There is a case to argue that most of us still *are* useless eaters... as long as we play our part, mindlessly consuming fake food, fake news, and fake entertainment within a giant, polluting, soulless System.

At the same time, the rhetoric espousing a harmonious future in which humanity lives in balance with nature has a certain appeal, but beneath it lurks a horrifying implication. It is possible that the Owners do envision a kind of idyllic Utopia... but only for themselves!

New breakthroughs in artificial intelligence and robotics may only leave the need for just enough other human beings to keep everything running. In the words of Klaus Schwab, when talking about his "Fourth Industrial Revolution" idea in September 2021, "Not everybody can be a robot polisher."

Ultimately, though, this is all just speculation. Whether the Owners want to wipe most of us out may not really matter. All we need to do is to look at what they are doing *right now*.

One thing we can say with confidence is, the System evidently does not care if we get sick, but in fact does clearly profit even more when we do. It is pushing terrible dietary advice in the face of all reason, other than its own short-term economic gain, and supports an industrial farming system that we can be confident will destroy most of the Earth's remaining arable soil within a few generations, even according to the UN's own Food and Agriculture Organization.

From those simple facts, we can make a few deductions.

First, the System has no issue lying to us. It has no problem with giving us entirely the wrong advice, even at the cost of our health, and also at the cost of our environment, the very earth beneath our feet.

Second, at the rate things are going, very soon the Earth is going to be unable to support a population anything close to today's 7.9 billion. So the point will be moot anyway.

That means the future of humanity really must not be a priority. Take time to let that sink in. In the pursuit of profit and power, the psychopathic System is ready to destroy much of the natural world along with its ability to support our current human population.

Whatever they call it—The Great Reset, the New World Order, Agenda 2030, the Fourth Industrial Revolution, or "Build Back Better"—all we really need to do is ignore the bullshit rhetoric, step back, and look at the bigger picture.

What does this future, which we are told is inevitable, *really look like*? Will it involve more government, or less? Will it allow us more freedom to choose, or less? And then there's the ultimate question: will it carry us back towards our ancestral tradition with our birthrights of harmonious living and vibrant health, or further away from it, with even more intensive lifestyles and increasing dependence on technology and the control of others? These are the questions that ought to keep us all awake at night.

And of course there is one other quite blatant feature of what they are telling us is an unavoidable future.

They are coming for the meat.

One more fact that "everyone knows" today is that we all need to eat less meat for the good of the planet. Wherever you look, you find the same message repeated.

In its video "8 predictions for the world in 2030" the World Economic Forum states:

"You will eat much less meat, an occasional treat not a staple, for the good of the environment and our health."

We can see the machinery already in motion, with nonprofit organizations and governments talking about putting new taxes on every pound of meat produced, imagining this will somehow be used to offset the "carbon cost" involved.

Of course we already know that the health argument is profoundly and entirely wrong. The weight of scientific evidence is so great that we must conclude the World Economic Forum is deliberately setting out to mislead on the health argument... But what about the environment?

The premise for the War on Meat is that we are currently engaged in killing the Earth through climate change, and that farming and eating meat play a significant role in that. Let's pick that premise apart and look at the facts.

We're going to invite you to take a further big step back and to consider the possibility of a whole new level of bullshit, which goes right to the core of their argument: We are killing the earth, and a major factor is *your* selfish beef-eating habit.

Why don't we take a moment to ponder that claim in the context of history.

Remember how we observed those who rule over society have always depended on the ever-present fear of some external threat, so that the people will demand protection, even at the price of their liberty.

Only recently, in the seventies and eighties, we were terrified the world was going to blow itself up. The US and USSR, we were told, had enough nukes to wipe out not just humanity but all large animal life for millennia. Now the nuke fear has largely gone away.

Then we were petrified of AIDS, but that didn't wipe us out either. And of course we then went on to face new, invisible threats from a series of novel viruses: Ebola, SARS, Zika, and most recently the COVID-19 family, which led to global lockdowns and demands for never-before-witnessed levels of mass social control.

Is there a pattern here? Constant threats of catastrophes whose most noticeable impact appears to be nothing more than *fear itself.*

And now they are telling you it's hamburgers! If you keep eating meat, we all face oblivion! The entire planet is in imminent danger and it's your fault, but you can gain absolution by putting different food on your plate.

Could this simply be the same old model: problem > reaction > solution?

When the godfather of Nazi propaganda, Hermann Göring, was asked how he managed to persuade the German people to accept the necessity of atrocities, his response was:

"...the people can always be brought to the bidding of the leaders. That is easy. All you have to do is tell them they are being attacked and denounce the pacifists for lack of patriotism and exposing the country to danger. It works the same way in any country."

What is unique about today's breed of existential problems is that they are *global and invisible*. Nuclear holocaust, viruses that do not respect borders, and now the imminent threat posed by cow burps.

In the modern day, we are even repeatedly reminded that each of us is responsible for *everyone on the planet*. That means you bear personal responsibility for billions of strangers, which is simply the old collectivism bullshit on a world-wide scale.

The Club of Rome is a think tank founded in 1968, shortly before the World Economic Forum, which describes itself as, "a platform of diverse thought leaders who identify holistic solutions to complex global issues and promote policy initiatives and action to enable humanity to emerge from multiple planetary emergencies."

The following passage comes from a book published by the Club of Rome in 1991 titled *The First Global Revolution*.

"The Common Enemy of Humanity Is Man

In searching for a new enemy to unite us, we came up with the idea that pollution, the threat of global warming, water shortages, famine and the like would fit the bill. In their totality and in their interactions these phenomena do constitute a common threat which demands the solidarity of all peoples. But in designating them as the enemy, we fall into the trap about which we have already warned, namely mistaking symptoms for causes. All these dangers are caused by human intervention and it is only through changed attitudes and behaviour that they can be overcome. The real enemy, then, is humanity itself."

The reframing is explained in clear language. Today's problems are *global* problems, and the common denominator is *us*. That insight suggests that perhaps the War on Meat could be hiding something even more insidious. Perhaps it is a front for a campaign against the human population.

It is of course conceivable that a strong argument could be made to force the world to change their diets to prevent climate catastrophe... if the assumptions were true! Let's continue to look at the facts.

As we have mentioned, the reality of the threat posed by beef depends on the following logic:

- First, the greatest threat to humanity's survival is climate change;

- second, that the climate change is caused by human activity;

- and finally that domestic animals play a significant enough part in that threat to warrant drastic action.

"Everyone knows" about the very real threat of climate change. The idea, which has wall-to-wall, 24/7 coverage, is that, since the Industrial Revolution, human activity has driven up the concentration of greenhouse gasses in the atmosphere, trapping more of the sun's energy and leading to a constant warming effect. The warming will in turn cause the collapse of the climate and lead to droughts, the melting of Arctic ice, and a rise in sea levels, among other horrors.

Interestingly, the emphasis has evolved in recent years. The phenomenon known as "climate change" used to be called "global warming", as we saw in the Club of Rome quote above from 1991. You can look up the relative popularity of the two terms using Google Trends, which will show that "climate change" overtook "global warming" as the preferred brand name around 2016.

One reason for this might be that the emphasis on "global warming" does not quite fit the evidence.

For example, something most people *do not know* is that, between 1940 and 1975, the world actually became progressively *colder*. This is despite the fact that industrial activity ramped up massively after the end of the Second World War. As a result, in the 1970s, the main climate story was the fear of global *cooling* and the prospect of an imminent ice age that could eliminate mankind!

Also, it should be noted that none of the warnings of doom and gloom have so far actually come to pass! In 1988, the New York Times gave the following ominous alert:

"If the current pace of the buildup of these gases continues, the effect is likely to be a warming of 3 to 9 degrees Fahrenheit [between now and] the year 2025 to 2050.... The rise in global temperature is predicted to ... caus[e] sea levels to rise by one to four feet by the middle of the next century." ~ Philip Shabecoff, *Global Warming Has Begun*

It hasn't happened. The sea levels have not risen, in fact the rich seem oblivious to the risk and have continued to invest in beachfront mansions.

In 2013 a leaked report from the International Panel on Climate Change revealed that global temperatures had only risen by a quarter of the amount they had predicted in 2007, constituting a "global warming pause". Bizarrely the report nevertheless concluded that the IPCC was now *even more confident* than before that global warming was both real and caused by human activity, raising their confidence level from 90% to 95%.

Overall, there has been an average temperature increase of only approximately 0.8° Celsius since the Industrial Revolution began, and most of that rise manifested prior to 1940. Put into the context of a much longer timeframe, that less-than-one-degree rise in temperature appears relatively insignificant. The world is cooler now than it has been for almost the *entirety* of the last nine and a half thousand years.

In the time of the Roman Empire, two thousand years ago, global temperatures were around one degree Celsius higher than today. In the time of the Ancient Egyptian civilization, which ended around 2500 years ago, temperatures were 2°C higher. Between five and nine thousand years ago, the Earth experienced a period called the Holocene Maximum, where temperatures around the world were estimated to have been somewhere between two and nine degrees Celsius higher than today.

Yes, we are currently seeing a modest rise in temperatures, but overall, the world is currently cooler than it has been at any time since the end of the last ice age and the entire span of the Holocene era... in other words the *whole of human civilization.*

Applying a little common sense, if humanity managed to thrive throughout that whole period, when temperatures were much higher than they are today, clearly nothing wiped us out.

The Paris Agreement, signed by most world governments in November 2016, set an overall target limit on average temperature increase to within two degrees Celsius above pre-industrial levels. Yet that would still be comfortably within humanity's normal range. So how would such a modest rise in temperature pose a cataclysmic threat to life now?

The next step in the climate change argument is that it is *human activity* that drives temperature changes. For now, let's ignore the three decades of cooling that occurred in the mid-twentieth century and accept the counter-argument that it was increased atmospheric pollution from factories and volcanoes that blocked out the sun's rays, which more than countered the supposed warming effect of all the greenhouse gasses.

Going back further in time, using data from ice cores, reveals a very consistent pattern of strong temperature fluctuations, which range from around four degrees Celsius higher to twelve degrees lower than the present day, driven by the Milankovitch cycle. In that big picture, we should now be around a temperature peak and should anticipate another sudden plunge sometime in the next few thousand years.

Until the past few hundred years, the Earth's human population was of course minimal, and yet the temperatures still varied widely between these predictable limits. If it wasn't our factories and our farting, burping livestock, what could possibly have driven this cycle?

It turns out that the most accurate predictor of global temperature changes is *solar activity*. In simple terms, when the sun is more active, the warmer the Earth gets. The explanation is that increased activity, which we can measure by the concentration of "sun spots", creates a solar wind as the sun throws particles out into space. These particles can interrupt cosmic rays, preventing them from entering the Earth's atmosphere, where they would normally interact with water vapor to form clouds. The more clouds, the less solar energy directly hits the Earth. The more solar activity, the fewer cosmic rays, resulting in less cloud cover, and the Earth heats up.

In fact, solar activity correlates almost exactly with historical global temperature fluctuations. But there is another problem with the hypothesis that higher carbon dioxide concentration drives the temperature up, which is that it appears to work *the other way round*.

Historical records show that, yes, atmospheric CO_2 does correlate fairly closely with temperature, but also that CO_2

increases occur *after* the temperature goes up, and likewise drops again following a period of cooling, with a consistent lag of several hundred years.

One explanation is that warmer temperatures on the land and in the sea stimulate the growth of plants and ocean-dwelling phytoplankton, which in turn feed more animal life, which then gives off more CO_2. Another is that the warmer sea water gets, the less dissolved gas it can hold.

Another likely factor that could also govern the world's temperature over a longer timespan, is changes in the Earth's orbit, in which our closest proximity to the sun varies according to a very long but predictable cycle.

Whichever factor, or combination of factors, are at play, at some times in the past, atmospheric CO_2 levels have clearly been three or more times higher than they are today.

Far from destroying life on Earth, higher CO_2 seems in fact to stimulate plant life, for the same reason commercial growers often pump CO_2 into their greenhouses to increase yields. We can see some modest level of the effect today because the world is in fact currently going through a period of getting greener.

Despite all those evident facts, authorities such as NASA and the UN's International Panel on Climate Change (IPCC) continue to state categorically that it is human activity that will destroy the planet. The NASA website proclaims that "the vast majority of actively publishing climate scientists - 97 percent - agree that humans are causing global warming and climate change." This is a disingenuous claim, as it came from an analysis of published papers that excluded the vast majority of papers that expressed no firm opinion either for or against human involvement, yet it continues to be repeated as fact by numerous politicians. The IPCC has also been guilty of inflating the perceived support in the scientific community by including on its reports the names of climate scientists who disagreed so strongly with the conclusions that they asked their names to be removed from the list of authors.

In summary, we can reduce the whole man-made-climate-change argument to one simple observation. Even if human activity *is* having some effect on the concentrations of certain atmospheric gasses, and even if those concentrations *will* lead to a warming effect, a resultant two- or three- or even four-degree increase in average temperatures still remains squarely within the normal range of historical human experience. (However, if it is true that the sun's activity is the major factor, we are more likely soon to enter another ice age.)

Now let's turn to the final piece of the argument that claims to prove why you *must* switch your steak for plant-based alternatives: How cows are a major cause of greenhouse gas emissions.

In 2006, the Food and Agriculture Organization of the United Nations released a report titled *Livestock's Long Shadow: Environmental Issues and Options*. It made shocking reading, with the headline claim that domestic animals contribute 18% of *all* anthropogenic greenhouse gas emissions. A later report, *Tackling Climate Change Through Livestock*, reduced that estimate somewhat to 14.5%. However, the methodology of both reports has been discredited, as they included recent short-term destruction of rainforests in their figures, dramatically bumping up the numbers. They also claimed that methane is a dangerously potent greenhouse gas while ignoring the fact that atmospheric methane is completely broken down after just ten years.

These UN reports continue to circulate, in much the same way that Ancel Keys' shoddy diet science from the mid-twentieth century never seems to go away, and probably for the same reason... because they suit the narrative. Countless papers and articles have been written on the subject of livestock and global warming, arguing the relative evils of methane versus carbon dioxide, and it seems as though the argument will rage on for some time, but we believe the whole issue can be resolved, yet again, with the simple application of common sense.

A few hundred years ago, prior to the arrival of the Europeans, it is estimated that there were between thirty and sixty million bison roaming the North American plains, resulting in deep, lush, rich soil (which coincidentally also happened to lock up huge amounts of carbon). Today, there are around forty million beef and dairy cattle combined in the United States. Considering bison are around double the size of domestic cattle, we can say the overall biomass of ruminants has not increased in the past few centuries.

In fact, we can state that the number of large ruminants the Earth supports has always been approximately the same: *as many as it could support!* That is the way nature works. The normal distribution model will always allow a species to expand its range and numbers according to, and up to the limit of, available resources. It really is that simple.

Now ask yourself, if all those grazing ruminants did not destroy the planet *then*, why are they blamed *now*? How did cows only start killing the planet in recent years? The argument simply does not make sense.

We can summarize that there is no clear-cut case that livestock are polluting the atmosphere, nor that these gasses are going to change global temperatures, nor even that an increase in temperature would be a problem for our continued existence.

So if the problem is not as bad as it is made out to be, why would we be told a lie?

The most likely answer must be to cause a reaction that will lead to a solution… but one that serves the Owners.

The level of climate crisis panic is incredibly high in our children's schools, in the media, in scientific literature, and not least in the halls of our governments. The perceived threat level is so high that people are taking to the streets and demanding action from their leaders. In fact, we are told that the problem is so great that it demands action that extends beyond even the reach of nations.

In November 2021, then-Prince Charles addressed the COP26 climate conference in Glasgow, claiming that the only way the world could face the climate threat was with a "vast military-style campaign" that would combine the resources of governments and the private sector and bring about what he called a "fundamental economic transition".

This is what it is all about, another final shift in power from the People to the Owners. And clearly they do not want us to go on eating meat.

The simple, biological facts are these. Eating the meat and fat of ruminant animals has always supported optimal human health. Eating meat and fat helps protect us from chronic disease. Eating meat and fat makes us stronger and smarter. Eating meat and fat means we are less addicted and less dependent on constant consumption.

Slave food does the opposite, leaving us sick, vulnerable, dependent, weak, and feeble-minded. Slave food has always made us easier to control, or to eliminate.

Another major factor is that the System abhors the natural, because it cannot *own it*. The first industrialists required intellectual property laws to protect the profits from the inventions they owned. Now, the same applies to the food on the shelves. Nothing made by nature can be patented, so we have been given brand new things to eat, reconstituted to original designs out of crude, basic ingredients and spat off industrial production lines by the millions. That's what's good for profits.

So it seems we have been sold several huge lies. Eating meat will not only kill you, but the planet too.

And the Owners must know this. They know they can lie, and they know they will get away with it as long as the People continue to believe what they are told.

"His primary rules were: never allow the public to cool off; never admit a fault or wrong; never concede that there may be some good in your enemy; never leave room for alternatives; never accept blame; concentrate on one enemy at a time and blame him for everything that goes wrong; people will believe a big lie sooner than a little one; and if you repeat it frequently enough people will sooner or later believe it."

That passage is from a psychological profile of a successful liar named Adolf Hitler.

The process is now almost complete. We are indoctrinated that every one of us has been born into a new kind of Original Sin, one in which we are automatically at fault. Now we are no longer responsible for ourselves and our loved ones, but for the whole human race, and even for the entire Planet Earth.

It is *your fault* that we are all facing an imminent disaster, not the corporations that burn the forests and strip-mine for minerals.

So you, the People, must repent. You must mend your ways, hand over your steak knives and switch to eating plants.

You will be happy to comply when your COVID vaccine passport transforms into the new "green passport", safe in the certain knowledge that it is all for the greater good.

When the robot checkout in the grocery store flashes red to indicate you have exceeded your individual monthly carbon-credit-controlled allowance for meat, you will be happy to swap the steak for a branded, patented, lab-grown alternative.

Whatever problems you may face in the future, our one world government will be there to save you. One other thing you can be sure of... the solutions will be patented.

But don't worry. In this future, you will own nothing, and you will be happy.

Chapter 17:
The Real Atrocity

"Formerly there were those who said: You believe things that are incomprehensible, inconsistent, impossible because we have commanded you to believe them; go then and do what is unjust because we command it.

Such people show admirable reasoning… Truly, whoever can make you believe absurdities can make you commit atrocities.

If the God-given understanding of your mind does not resist a demand to believe what is impossible, then you will not resist a demand to do wrong to that God-given sense of justice in your heart. As soon as one faculty of your soul has been dominated, other faculties will follow as well."

~ Voltaire, *Questions sur les Miracles* (1765)

As Voltaire warned centuries ago, our whole society has been led to believe things that are incomprehensible, inconsistent, and impossible. George Carlin colorfully highlighted the sheer ridiculousness of the crusade we are told we must all join today...

"We're so self-important! And the greatest arrogance of all, 'Save the planet!' What?! Are these fucking people kidding me?! Save the planet?! We don't even know how to take care of ourselves yet! We haven't learned how to care for one another and we're gonna save the fucking planet?!" ~ George Carlin

While that is an insult to our intelligence, it is not the real evil. Because we have been indoctrinated to believe absurdities, we have also found ourselves playing our part in a far greater atrocity, one that is being inflicted both against the human race and against nature itself.

It is necessary to take a long, hard look at the war on meat, to expose it for the absurdity it really is, because behind it lurks a far more insidious violation.

You have been told to believe the impossible: that *animal life* is playing a significant part in the destruction of the equilibrium of the whole climate, and could in turn pose a risk to life on Earth. Read that sentence as many times as you need to.

The System would have you believe the bullshit story that humanity is somehow independent from nature and that our ancestral diet is just some inconvenient evolutionary legacy. But it's okay because now we are fortunate to have wonderful new food choices that are "better for the planet". The System reassures you that, if you prefer not to eat meat in order to save the world, no problem! Instead you can choose a fake "beef" burger reconstituted from soy and pea protein isolate combined with dozens of other unrecognizable ingredients. That is what we are told the Earth needs now.

We already know this cannot be the case. To meet all your nutritional needs from a diet based mainly on corn, wheat, soy, sugar, and industrial seed oils is a mathematical impossibility. We know that nothing can support optimal health in the way that meat and fat can, so if we continue to consume what we are told to consume we will inevitably continue to be feebler, more dependent, addicted, sicker, and spending more on medicines than we do on food. (In the early 1970s, American families spent about twice as much of their household incomes on food that they spent on healthcare. Today that has done a total flip, with Americans now spending twice as much on health as on food.)

We also know that it is annual plant agriculture, not animal husbandry, that is responsible for the destruction of ecosystems all across the world. That fact has been proven time and time again over the span of human civilization.

The great paradox, which we cannot stress strongly enough, is that, far from being the problem, animals are actually a major part of the *solution*, whereas in fact the *real problem* we should be worried about is the *solution* they are trying to force on us!

We are being educated that the only answer to the world's predicament is a new and improved universal System in which the actions and freedoms of each citizen can be centrally monitored and controlled. The premise is that we must keep a lid on our wicked carbon emissions, despite the fact that the level of atmospheric carbon is a fraction of what it has been in the past (without suffocating life on Earth), *and* the average temperature is currently lower than it has been throughout almost the entire span of time since humans first settled and started to farm.

To appreciate fully the scale of the true atrocity behind the War on Meat, it is necessary to go back again to first principles, to look at the way nature works, and in particular how the elements of life are continuously cycled and recycled. Appreciating this perfect model, and how it is intrinsic to the natural world, will help expose the true atrocity that is being perpetrated.

In this chapter, we will focus on beef cattle as our case study, as they have been particularly singled out in the War on Meat.

Looking at the big picture, we can observe that it is always nature's tendency to create rich, deep, abundant, beautiful variety. We know that is a fact for the simple reason that it is what we observe around us, wherever nature is left to follow its own laws and build its own systems without man's interference.

In any ecosystem nature will always produce a wide variety of plant life that lives off organic matter, sunlight, water, minerals, and carbon dioxide. And animals will then inevitably proceed to fill the role of consuming that plant life, developing a range of ways to extract from plants what they need to build and power their bodies.

Other animals, the predators and scavengers, then come along to eat the animals that eat the plants. Carnivores have developed different ways of obtaining the energy and body-building nutrients they need, which come from their prey. As previously established, that is humans' place in the food chain.

But the food chain is not the way it is often presented from the anthropocentric perspective: as a hierarchical pyramid with predatory carnivores sitting at the top. The chain actually takes the form of a continuous *ring*, because whenever any animal dies, from the smallest nematode worm to a blue whale, it always creates food for a host of other life forms including bacteria, archaea, fungi, plants, and other animals. The same goes for plants and every other type of lifeform. The death of any living thing always creates the possibility of food for other life. In this way, the cycle of life truly has no beginning and no end.

Life depends on three fundamental factors: energy, water, and nutrients (which include carbon, nitrogen, and all the other building blocks needed to create living things). All energy originates from the sun, and all water cycles continuously around the air, waterways, oceans, ice, and land. For this case study, we will focus in particular on the third factor, the cycle of nutrients.

On land, the soil is nature's great nutrient store. For every life there always follows one inevitable death and all lifeforms must eventually return to the soil to be recycled into new plant, fungal, microbial, and animal life. Humans are no exception to this law of nature, which is why many in the Western world say, "Ashes to ashes, dust to dust," when we bury our dead.

However, the *scale* of abundance in this great cycle *is* highly variable, and it all starts with the soil. Wherever soil is destroyed, reduced to dirt, or blown or washed away to leave bare rock or sand, life cannot flourish. If the soil is stripped away, the amplitude of natural life cycles diminishes.

But wherever the soil is rich and deep, cool and moist, shielded from the elements by its vital blanket of constantly decomposing organic matter, life explodes in glorious richness and abundance. When the plant kingdom is provided with the right conditions to burst forth, the greening that results creates a cooling effect, which stimulates precipitation, in turn promoting further profusion of plant and animal life.

Although the Earth has experienced massive fluctuations in temperature throughout its history, the soil has nevertheless always been able to support life. As we have seen, soils are made up of far more than inert minerals, but are in fact extraordinarily complex ecosystems in which plant, fungal, animal, and microbial life coexist in a web of symbiotic relationships.

Because in nature everything is connected, the life above soil also plays a critical role in its health. And across much of the land today, it turns out that grazing animals are the key both to the soil's development and to its vitality. This stands to reason when you appreciate the fundamental symbiotic nature of all things. Grassland and grazers evolved together and therefore must logically depend on each other.

Many eons ago, the surface of the Earth was dominated by forests and the large plant-eaters were *browsers*, munching on trees and shrubs. Scientists believe that, around 65-50 million years ago, the Earth's temperature peaked at a massive 10-14°C warmer than it is today, and the land's surface began to dry out.

This is also around the time the dinosaurs are thought to have gone extinct.

The drier conditions meant some of the forests, which depended on a steady water supply, gave way over time to a totally new form of smaller, simpler, fast-growing plants: the grasses, which have the advantage of being able to adapt far more easily to drier conditions. Grass plants have the ability to respond rapidly to environmental changes, slowing down or speeding up their growth according to the availability of resources.

Today somewhere up to forty percent of the land on Earth is grassland of one sort or another, from prairie to steppe to savanna. Because nature always finds a solution that maximizes the range and abundance of life, the emergence of grasses gave rise to the evolution of new species of animals that specialized in grazing on grass. As is nature's way, the two depend on each other. In fact you cannot have optimum fertility on grassland *without* grazing animals, because they play a unique and vital role in both stimulating plant growth and accelerating the soil-building process.

Grass plants tend to remain upright when they die, which means they do not decompose rapidly. This is one way in which grazing animals play a key role. Without herds of large grazers, grassland soil would develop very slowly. But the passage of grazing animals helps trample dead grass onto the surface, where it can decompose more rapidly in the presence of water, fungi, and bacteria.

Frequent grazing also helps to keep grasses in their most active growth phase. Imagine that a grass plant's growth profile follows an S-shaped curve. If its leaves are cut too close to the surface of the soil, it will not be able to absorb much energy from the sun, and so can only grow slowly. As it puts out longer leaves, it will access more solar energy and build new roots, enabling it to grow as rapidly as possible until it reaches its full height, at which point growth slows and halts.

Optimal growth is therefore maintained if the grass is regularly grazed, meaning it does not top out at full height, but critically if it is also not over-grazed too close to the ground. Additionally, if a grass plant is cut down too far and too frequently, it will go into survival mode, sloughing off roots in order to help it survive what it perceives as a period of drought.

It used to be believed that overgrazing or overbrowsing by animals was a problem in drier climates, leading to desertification. That changed due to the research of another outlier.

In Southern Africa in the 1960s a young ecologist called Allan Savory was employed to participate in massive culls of elephant herds, in order supposedly to protect the rangelands from overgrazing. In total up to forty thousand elephants are believed to have been exterminated. However, when it transpired that the vegetation in fact *further deteriorated* after the removal of the elephants, Savory was devastated and dedicated himself to exploring the relationship between herds of herbivores and the vegetation they consume.

What Savory discovered through careful observation of nature's patterns radically challenged the science of the day. Rather than accelerating desertification, he realized that grazing actually did the opposite, helping to halt or even reverse the process.

Savory's major insight was that it was not so much the presence of large herbivores, or even their numbers on the land, but their *pattern* of movement and grazing that is the key to building soil efficiently. As always, the answer had been there all along, observable in nature's perfect systems.

Wherever you go in the world, herds of grazing animals adopt a similar pattern of behavior, moving together in tight groups to provide protection against predators. That necessarily means that each patch of land they graze will soon become covered in dung, and therefore the herd must keep moving on. As the herd moves away, the newly-fertilized grass is left to regrow, until it is grazed again some time later.

Another key factor is that larger herbivores do not nibble the grass right down to the roots, as sheep and goats might. Cattle wrap their tongues around a bunch of grass and rip off the top portion. Other large grazers such as horses use their powerful lips to pull at the leaves. As a result, regularly grazed grass plants are kept in the steep, fastest-growing portion of their growth curve until the next herd comes along.

Grasses, like many other plants, have special relationships with particular species of fungi, called mycorrhizae, which attach to the plant's roots and help supply nutrients from the soil. In return, the plant's roots exude sugars to feed the mycorrhizal fungi, which constitutes a significant component in the soil building process and also happens to sequester large amounts of carbon into the ground.

In this way, the influence of large ruminants accelerates the life cycle of grasslands and their soils. Their frequent-but-partial eating patterns keep the grass growing fast, and the liberal application of excrement recycles nutrients and organic matter back into the earth, with the help of legions of tinier animals such as dung beetles.

But that is not the whole picture. What if nature just stopped there? What would happen if herds of herbivores were just left to graze in peace, with no danger from predators? As it happens, we do have a case study that shows exactly what results.

Oostvaardersplassen is a 56-square-kilometer nature reserve set up in the 1980s in the Netherlands, in which animals are free to roam entirely as they wish, safe from predation. Here, a local resident describes how it works out.

"This piece of land holds, amongst others, thousands of red deer, Polish feral horses called Koniks, and feral cattle. These populations aren't managed and there are no large predators. Every winter thousands of these animals die slowly of starvation. The stench of the carcasses even makes people gag in the cities downwind. Every well thinking person wants these populations managed, in other words, limit the population to a level the land can sustain. However, the green mafia objects to shooting the surplus and thus the gruesome torment continues year after year."

The clear lesson is that, without population control, herbivores will breed too freely, expand rapidly in numbers, and overgraze the vegetation, which leads to inevitable starvation, and that actually results in a net *reduction* in life. Removing the predators seems to break nature's cycle.

The conclusion is that you cannot have optimally abundant grasslands without herds. But you also cannot have the herds without predators to keep them moving in a natural pattern and control their numbers and prevent destruction of the habitat.

In Zimbabwe Allan Savory experimented with mimicking the pattern of herd movement that he observed in nature by using local herdsmen to move their cows frequently in close mobs. What he discovered was that previously arid soil rapidly became richer in organic material and therefore able to hold more water, which in turn supported more plant life.

His years of research in the field led him to go on to establish the Savory Institute, which now supports farmers worldwide to rebuild soil and lush ecosystems, using as a primary tool the careful management of herds of grazing animals, and that helped to give rise to the modern *regenerative agriculture* movement, whose aim is to raise food in a way that positively *builds soil* instead of destroying it.

In regenerative agriculture it is human management, rather than the threat of predation, that keeps herds moving in natural patterns. However, that is only really feasible if humans also take on the predator's other key role, which is culling the herds to prevent overpopulation.

That is how nature's laws work, maintaining the flow of resources in perpetual balance in a way that also continuously generates variety and richness. The crucial factor is to *maximize* the cyclical movement of energy, water, and nutrients through the complex web of life. The more abundant the life and the more levels of living things in any ecosystem, the greater the cycling of resources.

Life and the cycle of resources are inseparable, constituting both cause and effect, according to nature's laws. This insight is key to understanding the real atrocity.

Humans' traditional farming methods, however, do not conform to nature's laws. In the name of efficiency, man has turned away from natural, rich, multi-layered ecosystems in favor of reductionism and the one-way flow of resources. So we cleared our fields of inconvenient life forms, including rodents, insects, and other plant species, to give way to monocrops. We also found it was more profitable to move cattle and other animals into confined areas and to fatten them up rapidly on a diet of grains.

Whereas nature's laws favor cycles and balance, man's System promotes hierarchies and imbalance, and you can trace it all the way back to the original bullshit: the invention of the idea that the land belongs to us.

But let's dig deeper and look again at another crucial way in which the soil beneath grasslands builds under natural conditions. Soil is largely made up of decomposing organic matter combined with mineral content, as well as water and a plethora of plant, animal, fungal, and microbial life. The organic matter comes from the huge array of living things that dwell both above the soil as well as in its top few feet.

Soil's mineral content, however, originates from below, being raised up by the gradual breaking down of the bedrock into subsoil, which then gets mixed into the topsoil by the actions of deep-growing plant roots, fungal networks, and burrowing animals. Each growing season, perennial plants can send their roots deeper and deeper underground to tap into the minerals held there, which will then be recycled into the humus when the plants shed leaves, die, or are converted into manure.

From this, we can see that the ideal scenario for an abundant and healthy biosphere is one that features a mix of permanent, perennial vegetation, which might include trees, shrubs, and perennial grasses, along with opportunistic annual plants that occupy any empty spaces. Some perennial grasses such as fescue can send their roots as far as five feet or more below the ground.

A wide range of healthy plant life will always naturally support a healthy herbivore population. In the wild, no large herbivore will ever eat grass exclusively. Given the opportunity, they will forage on a wide variety of plants, which may include grasses alongside other leafy low-growing herbs called forbs, the leaves of shrubs and trees, and even mosses and lichens.

In that way, they can listen to their bodies' signals, which will lead them instinctively to seek out specific foods that can provide whatever minerals and vitamins may be needed, thereby helping the animal to maintain optimal health.

Carnivorous animals, of course, lack the ability to convert plant matter like cellulose into amino acids and fatty acids. But they can still *inherit* full healthfulness by eating the meat and fat of nutrient-balanced herbivores. And, as we have seen, they in turn also provide an important role in keeping the herbivore populations in balance. Every animal's nitrogen-rich dung and urine are returned to the soil, along with the remains of their bodies after death.

From this you can get a picture of how nature always finds a way to fill any empty niche to create complete systems, where nutrients, energy, carbon, nitrogen, and water cycle constantly. The result is an incomprehensibly complex *food web*, in which no living thing exists in isolation, but is linked to countless others.

Let's contrast this with the model that man has developed to produce our food, which prioritizes profit over sustainability.

Agricultural soil that only supports monocrops of *annual* grasses, grains, or vegetables simply cannot maintain a healthy state in the long term, not only because of the destructive action of the plow, but also because shallow-rooted annuals will never reach down far enough to draw new minerals from deep underground up to the surface, nor help to penetrate and break up the subsoil. That's why soil that is constantly used for annual crops does not just quickly become devoid of organic life, but eventually of mineral content as well.

So the inevitable outcome of basing our food system primarily on annual plants, including the corn, wheat, rice, soybeans, and oilseed crops that form the majority of the modern human diet, is that minerals remain locked underground, and therefore never enter the food chain. Of course, if the soil becomes depleted of nutrients, the same will inevitably apply to the plants that grow on it.

We are told that animal farming is killing the planet, but in fact it is *annuals*, not animals, that are the real problem.

How does the System deal with the endemic problem of progressive loss of nutrients? By ignoring the problem and papering over it! When your only concern is maximizing profit, the *appearance* of healthfulness takes precedence over real, sustainable health.

After World War II, the United States was left with redundant munitions factories originally set up to create explosives. It turned out that it was relatively easy to convert these over to the manufacture of nitrogen-based fertilizers, which helped power the new Green Revolution that began in the 1950s. Simply spreading artificial fertilizers onto the land helped annual crops to grow fast, even miraculously in poor soils that lacked natural sources of nitrogen.

However the word "fertilizer" is completely inaccurate. The addition of these chemicals does not make soil more fertile, but less! What they do is effectively force crops to grow in poor soils where they normally might struggle, so the soil ends up losing what few minerals it still contains. The end result is produce that only has the *appearance* of vitality, based on faulty accounting that prioritizes calories produced per acre over real nutrition. And that is a recurring theme in the modern feed system.

Even though modern agriculture can continue to reap harvests with the support of artificial nitrogen, modern fruits and vegetables are becoming evermore depleted of real nutrition. Speak to anyone who grows heritage varieties of plant crops using organic methods, including no-dig gardening and permaculture, and they will tell you how the taste of naturally-grown fruit and vegetables is a world apart from what you buy in the stores. The simple reason is the vast difference in soil health.

In "A study on the mineral depletion of the foods available to us as a nation over the period 1940 to 1991", David Thomas took the results of a 1940 study in Britain that analyzed the mineral content of various plant foods and compared them to the equivalents in 1991. He found…

- Copper declined by 76%
- Calcium declined by 46%
- Iron declined by 27%
- Magnesium declined by 24%
- Potassium declined by 16%

It stands to reason that the loss of soil nutrients must also have some knock-on detrimental effect on the meat we raise. In fact, David Thomas also applied his tests to a range of meats, finding that, on average…

- Copper had declined by 24%
- Calcium by 41%
- Iron by 54%
- Magnesium by 10%
- Potassium by 16%

The startling conclusion is that you would need to eat twice as much meat, three times as much fruit, and between four and five times more vegetables to get the same amount of nutrients as you would in 1940.

Instead of allowing our animals to browse according to their natural instincts, the modern food System locks them up and force-feeds them grains, soybeans, and various agricultural byproducts. That imbalanced feed mix makes them quickly put on fat, facilitating earlier slaughter, which of course is good for profits, but not good for the animal's health... or the health of anyone who eats its meat.

Factory farming of animals has also achieved another remarkable feat, which is to convert the perfect natural fertilizer—animal dung—into an ecological hazard. Keeping animals in high concentrations means too much manure in one place, which must be disposed of, often either in waterways or in stinking man-made lagoons.

In the United States, the majority of beef comes from animals that have spent the first portion of their lives on permanent pasture, close to their ideal environment, and which are then finished for their last few months on grain and other feedstuffs in concentrated animal feeding operations.

If the System could, it would put cattle straight onto grains, but that is not economically viable as they would simply get sick and die before reaching viable slaughter weight. Nevertheless, even spending just a few months on non-species-appropriate feed, they must be given antibiotics, hormones, and other medications to strike a profitable balance, keeping them alive and looking healthy enough until slaughter.

So, while not ideal, US beef is still one of the healthier dietary options, and certainly preferable to consuming foods made from annual crops that have been grown on depleted soils.

However, factory-farmed hogs and poultry, which would naturally scratch and dig in the soil to meet their varied, omnivorous dietary requirements, tend to be fed exclusively on modern crops and their byproducts, so their meat and eggs will inherit any lack of minerals in the soil.

What does this mean for our health? Consumers who dutifully follow official guidelines and abstain from a high proportion of meat raised under natural conditions are doomed to suffer the same fate as the agricultural soils that become more devoid of nutrients with each harvest.

The truth is that our chronic health collapse is due to two primary factors: toxicity, and nutrient deficiency. We have already looked at the toxic and anti-nutritious properties of seed oils, sugar, and grains. But there is also a massive amount of evidence pointing to the impact of nutrient deficiencies all around the world.

Almost a century ago, Weston Price warned that the physical degeneration he observed on his extensive travels clearly resulted from nutrient deficiency, and yet nothing has been done about it. Instead the developed world has doubled down once again, churning out as many calories as possible without consideration to nutrient content.

Today at least two billion people around the world suffer from micronutrient deficiencies, that's one in four human beings on Earth. Over 150 million children under the age of five suffer from stunted growth and there is a statistically-relevant inverse correlation between impaired growth in children and the proportion of animal-sourced foods in a nation's diet. The micronutrients most often lacking in the predominantly plant-based diets of the world's poorest are vitamin A, vitamin B-12, riboflavin, calcium, iron and zinc... all of which are readily available in foods from animal sources.

So we have seen that the modern food System, with its emphasis on profitable annual row crops, is not only physically destroying the earth but is also leaving whatever soil remains depleted of nutrition. The plants that grow on such poor soil have less vitality with every harvest, and animals that are fed on annual crops inherit their poor nutrient content.

And the shortfall is passed on to humans, who are now suffering the effects of malnutrition en masse, and not only in less wealthy countries. According to a recent study, 31% of the U.S. population is at risk from at least one vitamin deficiency or anemia, 95% of adults and 98% of teens do not get enough vitamin D, while 61% of adults and 90% of teens are lacking in magnesium.

The reality is that *every* part of the modern food system now adheres to the factory-farming model: not just the animals, but the crops and even the soil itself, and it is all down to the parasitical, psychopathic accounting model built into the System.

In nature, the constant sustainable cycling of energy, water, and nutrients ensures that health is *intrinsic*, and generates more life. But in our industrial feed System, the cycles have been broken. The endless succession of annual crops cannot build soil as fast as the plows can destroy it. Our fields continue, for the time being at least, to deliver an abundance of calories but with diminishing nutritional value.

In the System the surface *appearance of health* is all that matters. So we spray the land with artificial, petrochemical-based fertilizers, and pump the animals with hormones and antibiotics. If the fruits and vegetables are plump and sweet, they will sell. If the meat looks fatty and pink, due to the addition of nitrites or sulfites, shoppers will buy it. The uninformed consumer cannot see the invisible nutrient content, or lack of it.

The net result is that the last life has almost been sucked out of our farmland, and what remains is also running very low! Our most immediate and undeniable threat is not climate change, but the loss of topsoil. We *are* literally losing the Earth! Agricultural soil is being evaporated or washed into our rivers and oceans at an alarming rate: twenty-three billion tons every year, that's one percent of all the Earth's topsoil every twelve months. It is easy to see that most of it will be gone within a few generations.

But that in itself, while tragic and appalling, is not the real atrocity, which runs even deeper than the chronic degeneration in physical health. And it all points back to the unnatural, corrupt accounting model that the System is built on.

By placing value only on how much it can *extract*, without regard for what needs to be put back, the soil on which all life on land depends has degenerated catastrophically, and of course our health has inevitably followed suit.

But it does not end there. As shocking and as tragic the degeneration of the land and our bodies may be, they are still only *symptoms* of the real atrocity, which is an insult to the most fundamental laws of nature. The slide into degeneration not only impacts our health and our future survival, but even our sense of self, what it *means to be human*.

For our illustration we chose to focus on the example of cattle on grassland, but could have used any natural system. The key realization we must emphasize is that, wherever you look in nature, every living thing is connected, everything is linked to everything else through a myriad of relationships.

Understanding the *nature* of those connections reveals the secrets of life, and the atrocity that the System truly represents.

The fundamental lesson we must learn from observing nature's patterns is that the cycle of nutrients, energy, and water is more than just essential to life... *it is life*!

Natural systems always give rise to the continual *generation* of life. Its endlessly flowing cycles create the possibility of abundance and richness everywhere and for every living thing. Creation works through flow, elegantly finding the balance between entropy and chaos.

This seemingly simple quote from one pioneer of ecological farming, Joel Salatin, provides another clue to understanding the essential role of food in life's eternal creative force.

"Everything in nature is eating and being eaten." ~ Joel Salatin

In nature, all life is food for other life. And the act of consumption is how life *works*. The motive to consume, in other words to cycle nutrients, is the imperative that drives all biological processes.

The pursuit of nourishment is the engine of life. It is the *why* of all life.

Plants *consume* sunlight, water, and minerals, so that they can reach maturity and reproduce, and they in turn become food for animals, fungi, and the plethora of life in the soil.

Bacteria and fungi do not just mechanically break down organic matter, they are following their genetic imperative to *consume* what they need.

Herbivores *consume* plants, which they convert into animal matter, often with the help of hosts of microorganisms, which in turn are also following their genetic drive to *consume*.

Carnivores *consume* herbivores, and they, in their turn, will become food for even more life.

"We are all tomorrow's food." ~ Ken Wilber

Once we truly appreciate this web of interconnectedness, the picture that emerges shows that the relationships that link all living things relate to the *search for sustenance*. The existence of life and the pursuit of food are inseparable. They are one and the same.

If we were to map out every living thing in creation, that map would take the form of a giant food web. In other words, you could say that every being's *place* in any ecosystem within the web of life is defined by what it consumes, and by what will eventually consume it.

The feeding relationships also reflect *how* an animal lives. Because the search for sustenance is what drives life, a being's place in the food web dictates its daily behavior, moving towards the things it needs to eat, and ideally avoiding those things that might want to eat it.

In fact, it could be said that a species' place in the food system has a more immutable significance within the web of life that persists beyond that species. For example, zebra browse bushes and graze grass on the African savanna, and their other primary survival concern is to avoid predation by lions. Now, if the zebra species were suddenly wiped out, another zebra-like species would soon arrive to fill the important gap left in the food web.

With this understanding, we can see that food is far more than a lifestyle choice, but rather it is definitive of a living organism and its proper place in the universe.

So, in pushing us to abandon our ancestral diet and to turn to plants, the System is not only encouraging the degeneration of our physical vitality and the land on which we live, but the decay of our very identity as human beings.

"Not to know one's true identity is to be a mad, disensouled thing—a golem. And, indeed, this image, sickeningly Orwellian, applies to the mass of human beings now living in the high-tech industrial democracies. Their authenticity lies in their ability to obey and follow mass style changes that are conveyed through the media. Immersed in junk food, trash media, and cryptofascist politics, they are condemned to toxic lives of low awareness. Sedated by the prescripted daily television fix, they are a living dead, lost to all but the act of consuming." ~ Terence McKenna

For countless generations of humans, food *was* life, it defined who we were and where we belonged. We didn't just hunt and gather, we *were* hunter-gatherers. That was the driving force behind our movements and our daily decisions.

Perhaps most profoundly, playing our designated role in the food web meant that we knew who we were and where we belonged, which was on the land.

With their tendency to balance and flow, the laws of creation cause life to generate. Man's System, however, only knows how to extract and channel resources in one direction, up the pyramid of power, and it will always result in degeneration.

So you might say the degeneration has extended to infect the human spirit. In losing our connection to our food and our place on the Earth, we have lost far more.

Perhaps that is the real reason why so many of us are bored, depressed, addicted, and violent. Is it that we have simply forgotten *who we are*?

If so, this System we have helped to create is truly a blasphemy against the human spirit, and it goes against the most fundamental, sacred laws of creation. *That* is the real atrocity that lurks behind the War on Meat.

Of course living in the fantasy that we somehow exist above nature does not mean we get to escape the reality of its fundamental laws. We cannot keep taking without putting back forever. Balance and order must and will eventually return.

The big question is, which way is balance going to be restored?

One solution could be if humanity were to wipe itself out, in which case the natural world will recover, as it always has.

Another possible path is the one that maintains the privilege of the Owners, but which may necessitate a large-scale depopulation, as the cryptic Georgia Guidestones commanded.

"Maintain humanity under 500,000,000 in perpetual balance with nature."

But could there be another way, one that does not require a mass cull of useless eaters? Is there still a chance for us to rediscover how to thrive on the Earth in harmony before it is too late?

We believe there is. There is a way back to claiming our birthright, to what it means to be human, and it all starts with restoring our relationship with food.

Chapter 18:
When Tyranny Becomes Law

The previous chapters have presented a version of the story of the human race leading from ancestral and ancient times up to the present day. If our narrative is tainted by one overarching feature, it is *degeneration*.

Straying ever further away from our connection with nature, most fundamentally through our relationship with food, has come at a great cost, and perhaps we have even forgotten what it means to be fully-evolved humans. Surely each of us knows in our heart and soul that the present state of the human race is somehow not the life we were born to experience.

Let us briefly review the evidence. The earliest incontrovertible signs of human degeneration came from the anthropologists who documented the clear physiological deterioration that occurred when we switched from hunting and gathering to farming crops, where we very rapidly lost stature as well as brain size. It is important to remember that even that change only occurred very recently, in evolutionary terms, somewhere between 20,000 and 1000 years ago depending on region, in other words only between *10% and 0.5%* of the generally accepted time that Homo sapiens has been walking the Earth.

In addition to physiological degeneration, we also have evidence showing a decline in healthfulness. Archeological records from the Ancient Egyptians and the Idaho study, among many others, indicate a stark increase in the prevalence of chronic diseases between hunter-gatherer and farming communities.

More recently, only in the last 150 years—that's less than *one thousandth* of our time here—human health took another dramatic plunge downward with the introduction of industrial farming and processing of crops, and the abomination that is ultra-processed food.

We then saw how, in the early twentieth century, Weston A. Price was in a unique position to compare the effects of these novel, processed food sources versus people's traditional diets side-by-side. The sudden negative impacts he documented on physiology, mental faculty, and chronic disease led him to issue a powerful warning about impending degeneration, which he concluded could only have come about as a direct result of dietary nutrient deficiencies.

Price's book also raised the obvious moral question, *"Is it just for society to permit production of physical and mental cripples?"* That question should quite rightly be at the front of our minds today, almost a century later, not to blame the victims, but to hold to account the decision makers who make our laws and set the guidelines.

It is now clear that Price's grim warnings, although published and widely available, have gone unheeded in the corridors of power. As a result the modern world would find itself bombarded with epidemics of many chronic illnesses that had previously been very rare, not least diabetes, heart disease, and cancer. While there have been perennial calls for more research, the quite basic and obvious causes that Weston Price and many other scientists have tried to draw attention to have been systematically ignored for decades by our leaders.

The only rational explanation we can draw, in the face of the overwhelming body of scientific evidence, is that those in charge must have given their blessing to the degeneration. It suits their objectives. Just as we saw in the chapter on slave food, these slave owners do not care about our long-term healthfulness and vitality… because there is more profit to be made when the population is unhappy and sick. To use Price's language, these people are guilty, at the very least, of permitting the crippling of the People.

In parallel with our own health collapse, we have also witnessed the ongoing catastrophic degeneration of much of the world's topsoil, as has been highlighted by David Montgomery and many others. It is estimated that, in the few thousand years since we started to till the earth, we have already lost up to one third of all arable land, but the destruction has accelerated so much since industrialization that another third is at risk of degradation by the end of the current century!

We should be in no doubt that the majority of the human race is facing a very real and imminent threat to its survival, a ticking time bomb, and it is not going on up in the air above our heads but beneath our feet.

What about society itself? Can we say that life is actually getting better from a socioeconomic perspective? When you consider that just fifty years ago most families could afford to buy their own home with only one adult going out to work it is clear that, for all our ideas of progress, today most of us seem to be working more yet seeing less benefit.

Do we need to ask who is enjoying the fruits of our labor? There can be no question that the wealth gap between the top few and the rest is greater than it has ever been, or that it continues to widen at a startling pace.

Has our mental health fared any better? Clearly that has gone the same way as the general collapse in health, with skyrocketing levels of diagnoses and antidepressant use. This can be explained in part by the many links that have been observed between poor diet and mental degeneration, including the numerous harmful effects of excess sugar as well as insufficient amounts of the healthy fatty acids required to support proper brain function.

But we should also ask whether the unprecedented levels of bullshit required to hold the facade of Society together must also take a heavy toll. Not only are we bombarded by more assaults against logic than ever, but today we are also led to believe that open thought and discussion are unacceptable. We are now not only told where we can and cannot go, what we can and cannot do, what we should or should not eat, what we may and may not say, but even what we can and cannot *think*! Can we really call this progress? How is the mind supposed to maintain its sanity in the face of this maelstrom of paradox?

We can also go further and consider the possibility of our emotional and even spiritual degeneration as a society. How has removing us from our place in the food web affected our fundamental *sense of self*?

As it happens, science offers further shocking evidence that depriving an animal of its species-appropriate diet and its naturally-ordained position in the web of life inevitably leads to multiple forms of degeneration. Here we will mention just three examples.

Between 1932 and 1942, Dr. Francis Pottenger, a contemporary of Weston Price's, ran what became known as the Pottenger Cat Study. He fed control groups of cats on raw meat, raw milk, and cod liver oil, while test groups were given a diet of pasteurized milk and cooked meat.

The results were alarming. The first generation of cats that had been fed on the processed feed started to develop allergies and skeletal deformities. Their offspring showed signs of organ degeneration, in particular glandular problems. The third generation suffered a range of degenerative diseases, while the fourth not only manifested mental disorders but also turned out to be infertile!

Pottenger's work reinforced Weston A. Price's findings in proving how rapidly degeneration can manifest. Note that, while Price's book was titled "Nutrition and Physical Degeneration", he also offered extensive comments on the marked decline in behavioral standards and social cohesion he observed in communities after the adoption of inappropriate, imported foodstuffs.

In the 1960s J. L. Kavanau carried out a series of experiments using white-footed mice. He noticed that mice that had been captured from the wild demonstrated significantly higher capability and interest in life compared to those bred in captivity. He remarked that trying to understand wild mice by studying the behavior of captive-bred mice was as much use as aliens landing in the grounds of a mental asylum and observing its inmates in order to learn about the human race!

Kavanau noted, "Many responses of small captive mammals cannot be interpreted at face value because of severe distortions of behavior that are caused by depriving the wild animal of natural outlets for activity." His experiments point to the importance of natural stimuli to an animal, and how removing day-to-day activities such as exploration and finding food can lead to a rapid degeneration both in mental faculty and in spirit.

Another very foreboding series of experiments was carried out by the behavioral researcher John B. Calhoun in the 1970s.

He placed breeding groups of mice and, later, rats into self-contained "utopian" environments that had been carefully designed to cater to all the animals' physical needs, with ample space, bedding, and a constant supply of food.

In every one of his experiments, Calhoun observed the same tragic pattern unfold. Initially the rodents would just multiply rapidly in number, but eventually every population started to manifest a range of bizarre behavioral patterns. These included mothers abandoning their young, some individuals losing interest in mating and instead being totally obsessed with self-grooming, while dominant males became prone to unprovoked violence, to raping females as well as other males, and even to cannibalism.

On the surface, it would appear that in all these experiments the rodent populations had no motive to engage in such self-destructive behaviors. After all, their full range of needs seemed to be met. Could it simply be that, in being provided with all the food and apparent comfort they could want, they somehow lost touch with their innate rodent instincts, the natural desire to explore the world in the search of sustenance?

We have to consider, if being removed from their place in the natural food web could have such shocking consequences for rodents, could modern humans also be suffering a similar fate? Could replacing the pursuit of real, species-appropriate food with picking "food-like products" off the grocery store shelves also be damaging *us* emotionally, socially, and spiritually?

Perhaps it is no wonder that so many of us feel a deep draw towards pursuits such as hunting, fishing, gardening, raising animals, and foraging... all activities that were associated for eons with sourcing our sustenance.

In summary, our premise is that, following the waves of rapid technological change, which have only come more frequently since the Industrial Revolution, we are now heading for oblivion. The human race is on board a bus that is not only speeding towards the canyon edge, but accelerating!

While outliers have tried to warn us time and time again across the generations, it is clear that their warnings have been systematically suppressed, leading up to this time, when we are surely witnessing the crunch point for humanity.

"Human beings, who are almost unique in having the ability to learn from the experience of others, are also remarkable for their apparent disinclination to do so." ~ Douglas Adams

Of course you will always be able to find plenty of evidence to counter all those outliers who have tried to warn us over the years... from Plato to Voltaire, Weston Price to Vilhjalmur Stefansson, David Montgomery, Zoë Harcombe, Allan Savory, and the countless others we cannot possibly mention. Discrediting voices of dissent is just one of the System's defense mechanisms.

On the other hand, if you choose to pay attention not only to the System-sanctioned, mainstream, orthodox science, you are free to make up your own mind and ask the pertinent question:

If the outliers were all telling the truth, what are the implications for us?

After all, if you cannot trust official guidance even on something as basic as what constitutes a suitable diet, what else can you—or can't you—trust? The implication is that our leaders cannot be relied on to put our welfare first... on any matter!

And, if that is the case, should we not dare to entertain the idea that the whole modern world, this System we grew up in, is intrinsically *hostile* to our well-being?

"A good tree cannot bring forth evil fruit, neither can a corrupt tree bring forth good fruit." ~ Matthew 7:18

That realization brings us to a critical pivot moment...

Red Pill or Blue Pill?

We may contend that the totality of the available evidence proves conclusively that the System, and the political leaders who make up its theatrical cast, cannot be trusted... but ultimately, as it affects how you live your life, the decision can only be yours alone.

You could choose to take the Blue Pill and continue in the belief that our governments, and the emerging World Government, are working in good faith in the best interests of everyone, striving to end world hunger and pursuing justice, prosperity, and freedom for all.

If you can find it in your heart to put your trust in the politicians, transnational corporations, and NGOs, then the Blue Pill is an option. Hold out for better leaders, if that is what feels right to you. If that is the case, you can stop reading now and consider giving this book to someone else.

However, if, based on all the evidence available to you, a Blue Pill existence is no longer a realistic choice, right now you very likely find yourself faced with some unsettling possibilities, the prospect of breaking out of decades of miseducation, and the uncertainty about what will replace it.

To entertain the idea of accepting that the world we have grown up in is built on a carefully crafted mythology designed to keep us separate from our true nature represents a profound, and possibly irreparable, cognitive break.

Nobody should underestimate the seriousness of that Red Pill fracture, of accepting that many of the most important things you have been told are true are in fact deliberate falsehoods, and all the subsequent ominous implications.

At this point you could be asking yourself how we got here, how this insane scenario could even be *possible*! If it seems totally nonsensical to you, good! That is a positive sign.

We believe there is a simple answer, which is that *the people in charge are not like us*. They *are* psychopaths, and their System *is* psychopathic.

When you consider the possibility that, because they believe they are superior, that they deserve to own everything, and that the rest of us are just pawns in their game, the world actually starts to make much more sense. Suddenly, looking at the words and actions of the tiny minority who run things will appear less incongruous... as crazy as it may all still appear.

And, make no mistake, it *is* crazy!

It's not you!

"Our society is run by insane people for insane objectives. I think we're being run by maniacs for maniacal ends and I think I'm liable to be put away as insane for expressing that. That's what's insane about it." ~ John Lennon

We can find some solace in accepting that it is simply the nature of the psychopath to keep on taking more and more until there is no more left to take. And perhaps we don't need to hate them for that, but simply observe it for what it is and then choose to apply our energy in more positive directions.

198

Maybe the Owners are doing it deliberately, or it could be they are totally stupid, or perhaps they simply do not care. Ultimately, it does not matter if they really want to kill us off (although there is plenty of documented evidence to support that), nor is it relevant whether their intention may be to do it within the next few years or over several decades. The bottom line is, we *are* headed for the end of days.

And furthermore we must maintain that, whether the Owners are mentally ill or not, this state of affairs, which we could trace all the way back to the first land ownership deeds, is profoundly immoral.

In the words of one eminent thinker...

"If people let government decide which foods they eat and medicines they take, their bodies will soon be in as sorry a state as are the souls of those who live under tyranny." ~ Thomas Jefferson

"Tyranny" may seem like a strong word, but we believe it applies accurately to our present situation. The following definition of the term has also been attributed to Jefferson: "Tyranny is defined as that which is legal for the government but illegal for the citizenry."

Is it legal for you or me to control another's thoughts, to feed them falsehoods that lead them unknowingly to poison their body? No, that would clearly constitute criminal abuse. So, if successive *governments* do the same to us, we are surely living in a state of tyranny. And if we are living under tyranny, then we have a moral responsibility to resist it.

The following passage from the English philosopher John Stuart Mill perfectly embodies the natural and inalienable rights of the individual according to the spirit of common law.

"...the only purpose for which power can be rightfully exercised over any member of a civilized community, against his will, is to prevent harm to others... In the part which merely concerns himself, his independence is, of right, absolute. Over himself, over his own body and mind, the individual is sovereign." ~ John Stuart Mill, On Liberty, 1859

In the final three chapters we will address the question of what each of us can do to remedy this situation. Or perhaps the correct question is, what *must* each of us do, because if what seems to be happening is real, it must be viewed as criminal, whether by intent or through negligence.

A strong case can also be made that conspiring to mislead with fatal consequences would also constitute one or more crimes against humanity. These are defined in the 1945 London Charter of the International Military Tribunal as, "Murder, extermination, enslavement, deportation, and other inhumane acts committed against any civilian population…"

Let us once again recall the moral dilemma that Weston A. Price raised almost a century ago: *"Is it just for society to permit production of physical and mental cripples?"* Surely the answer is resoundingly negative. This state of affairs must be seen as fundamentally unjust and unlawful.

If our leaders suppress the true science about the food we eat, permit and even actively promote through subsidies and miseducation the spread of toxic fake foodstuffs that lead to sickness and death, a case can be made that such actions constitute "murder, extermination, and enslavement", thereby meeting at least one definition of crimes against humanity! And if that is the case, are we therefore not morally bound to rebel?

The idea of standing up to unjust rule is no mere delusional fantasy, but a basic human obligation that has been advocated by some of our most respected political and philosophical thinkers.

"When tyranny becomes law, rebellion becomes duty." ~ Thomas Jefferson

"Civil disobedience becomes a sacred duty when the state has become lawless or corrupt." ~ Mahatma Gandhi

"{Our problem is not civil disobedience…} Our problem is civil *obedience*. Our problem is the numbers of people all over the world who have obeyed the dictates of the leaders of their government… and millions have been killed because of this obedience. Our problem is that people are obedient all over the world, in the face of poverty and starvation and stupidity, and war and cruelty. Our problem is that people are obedient while the jails are full of petty thieves, and all the while the grand thieves are running the country. That's our problem. We recognize this for Nazi Germany. We know that the problem there was obedience, that the people obeyed Hitler. People obeyed; that was wrong. They should have challenged, and they

200

should have resisted; and if we were only there, we would have showed them." ~ Howard Zinn, Voices of a People's History, 1970

Is this not one of those key moments in time when the human race *must* stand together and disobey? After all, it is our own lives that are at stake.

For our own sakes, and for the sake of humanity, we *have* to throw ourselves from the bus before it goes over the edge. We have to change things, there can be no other choice.

Of course the first step in overcoming any problem is to admit you have one. The next is to admit what role you may have played in creating it.

It might seem absurd to suggest that the 99.99% of us who are victims of the System have brought it upon ourselves, but it is a crucial step.

Consider that, from the Owners' psychopathic point of view, it is quite possible they believe they have done nothing wrong. They may think that the state of things is in fact perfectly justified, because, after all, the People allowed it to come about.

And they would be absolutely right!

The truth is we only have this System precisely *because* we have allowed it. *We* have let ourselves be bewitched by the soporific distractions of consumerism, obeyed the rules, chosen an easy and comfortable life... and all the time we have continued to degenerate as a race. We never noticed the creeping decay because our memories are short and because we have allowed our worldview to be dictated to us by the psychopaths in power instead of by our own elders.

However we account for it, the fact that we have allowed ourselves to forget our place in the natural world and to be conned into believing the System is real has come at a terrible cost. But the most important question now is not why or how it happened.

The narrative we have offered in this book presents one way to understand it. But, once we accept that it has only come about *because* we allowed it, just a single pertinent question remains: will we—can we *afford to*—*continue* to allow it?

If we are to cling on to any hope, our path to redemption can only begin with rejecting that this is the way the world must be, so that we can set about creating a new one.

But you might wonder, do we even have a choice? Can we even dream about changing the world we live in?

Actually, the answer is a resounding "Yes!" We *do* have a choice, we do have other options and alternative possible futures.

As we have established, both common sense and scientific evidence present a clear message that there is something very wrong about the situation we find ourselves living in today.

There can be no question about whether we can continue to allow psychopaths to rule our lives. If, as it appears, the present assault on the human race's health and spirit constitutes at the very least tyranny, or at worst actual crimes against humanity, we have not only a moral right, but a moral obligation, to resist it.

Make no mistake, for all its bullshit rhetoric about progress, we cannot wait for the System to fix itself. It cannot and will never work for the benefit of all. In fact, you could say the System is working just perfectly, according to its own insane, parasitical motives.

No, hoping and waiting for any kind of solution to come down from above is really just the System talking. Of course that message is deeply ingrained in our minds because we have been educated by that same System since birth. A better version of the System can never be the answer. Do not wait for the right politician to come into power, or for the United Nations and World Economic Forum to change their policies. We have already had countless generations of monarchs and politicians and business owners, and all the while our degeneration has gathered pace. A slightly better cast of frontmen is not going to solve our problems.

No, the solution can only come from the ground up, it can only start with us. A lot of us.

If we can no longer even entertain carrying on as things are, dutifully riding the bus as it careers toward the canyon edge, if the human race is to have a future, we are going to need to make some big changes.

The question we are all asking ourselves right now is *what* on earth we can do about our situation. In the final three chapters, we will look at a few simple and achievable ideas about how we might organize our lives differently.

Simply put, we have to turn things around. The word for turning a thing around is "revolution" and we must accept that it is the only real option left for humanity. The word "revolution" can also be defined as, *"a fundamental change in the way of thinking about or visualizing something,"* and also, *"the overthrow or renunciation of one government or ruler and the substitution of another by the governed"*. We feel both those aspects are pertinent.

If the fruits of the System over the past few thousand years have been degeneration, then our only path home must surely be one of *regeneration*.

We have to *regenerate*... our bodies and minds and spirits, along with our precious, natural home.

Our revolution can happen on three levels... We must first regenerate our minds; then regenerate our bodies and our health; and finally we may have a chance of regenerating our society and our world.

Chapter 19:
Revolution Part One: Your Mind

From birth all of us, the People, have been fed a constant diet of bullshit, both mentally and materially.

This is not acceptable.

We need a revolution, in both senses of the word, encompassing both a change of perspective and a change to the way we manage our society. The first part, perspective, is the focus of this chapter. In fact, you can be assured that the shift has already begun. Its seeds have already started to grow within you and countless others, and it is gathering pace.

Revolution must first happen at the individual level, and in fact it can *only* happen individually for each one of us. While we might yearn for a social revolution, there you find a kind of paradox at play. *If and when* enough of us achieve our own personal revolutions, it must inevitably also manifest at the societal level. However, if we wait for it to happen in society first, it will never happen.

So let us continue what has already begun.

The only place that our regeneration revolution can begin is in our own minds. We cannot hope to bring about real change in our personal wellbeing, our families, or our communities, unless we first reclaim the right to free thought, our innate, divinely-ordained mental sovereignty.

Thought always precedes manifestation. That is why we have focused on showing diet miseducation bullshit in this book, because before you can change your actions you must first change your beliefs.

We have to begin the process of mental liberation by admitting the uncomfortable truth that we have been complicit in our own enslavement. Only when we each admit that we are not in fact the victims but the *authors* of our present situation can we move forward to author a new experience of life.

While it may certainly be challenging to accept that we are largely responsible, it is double-edged, because taking ownership over our situation also means that the power to save ourselves must already be in our hands.

"Emancipate yourselves from mental slavery, none but ourselves can free our mind." ~ Bob Marley, Redemption Song

There is of course a basic physiological aspect to reclaiming your power to think, which is to allow your brain to function optimally. If your body is locked in a constant up-and-down pattern, battered by waves of sugar, insulin spikes, and incessant hunger, how can you perform anywhere close to your potential? Cutting out the slave food and instead fuelling your physical being with the healthy, energy-packed, nutrient-dense fats it needs will give you a noticeable boost in mental stability. Science is also discovering strong links between gut health and mental health, which is yet one more reason why adopting a species-appropriate diet is a key step to rediscovering your power.

With that out of the way, let us move on and reclaim ownership over our minds!

As we will show, the process is actually remarkably simple, but it does depend on taking a big step. It seems there is no middle ground; either the world is insane or we all are. When you peek behind the curtain, even something as apparently mundane as food reveals a System that can only be being "run by maniacs for maniacal ends" as John Lennon put it.

Once you take the step and accept that we have grown up in a maniacal world, you will be able to see through the bullshit, discover the great secret that we will reveal in this chapter, and only then be truly free.

The great secret is hidden in plain sight, in fact within the very nature of bullshit itself.

Ask yourself, why did bullshit ever come about in the first place? And why would more and more bullshit need to be manifested over time?

"An illusion it will be, so large, so vast it will escape their perception. Those who see it will be thought of as insane." ~ J. Michael Thomas Hays, *Rise of the New World Order: The Culling of Man*

From the outset, bullshit has existed for one main purpose: to create an illusion that seeks to draw attention away from the wealth gap between those who have the most resources and influence and those who have the least. That gap has had to keep widening over the years because it is the only way the Owners could maintain the illusion of their own superiority, and to protect themselves from the truth and its inevitable consequences.

That meant they had to keep finding new ways to put ever more distance between us and them, which is why we have been subjected to increasing layers of propaganda, bureaucracy, abstraction, miseducation, shady accounting, social power hierarchies, and all the other forms of falsehood.

If we look at that relentless expansion in the cold light of day, we notice a fundamental problem inherent with bullshit. Like any way of distorting reality, such as drugs or alcohol, make-up or plastic surgery… once you start it is easy to find yourself needing to use more, and more frequently!

"Oh, what a tangled web we weave, when first we practice to deceive!" ~ Sir Walter Scott

For sure, there is an incredible amount of bullshit around today. It is wall-to-wall, seeming to seep out of every screen and every speaker twenty-four hours a day, seven days a week… but of course sheer volume does not make a thing any more true.

In fact, it seems as though the bullshit has peaked since the advent of the Internet and social media. Now that every one of us can potentially be a reporter or news editor instead of just a passive consumer of news, the Owners have faced a counter-movement of citizen-powered journalism that threatens even their cherished mainstream media, which they bought at great expense.

"If you only knew how much money was spent to brainwash you, you would realize how special you are." ~ Anonymous

As we described in our first book, *The Red Pill Revolution (2021)*, we, the People, are beginning to find our voice once again, thanks in no small part to the democratizing power of social media. One by one, individuals are stepping out of the System and into their sovereign authority, reclaiming *their* right to decide what is right for them.

That is why even so-called "social" platforms are now actively censoring the expression of free speech. Today, if you disagree with the party line on a particular topic, you are labeled a dangerous science-denier or conspiracy theorist.

That's how you can see that bullshit is all they have! And when the wall of bullshit starts to split and crack, all they can do is apply even more bullshit. As more of us wake up and realize just how deeply we have been conned, the more the System has to double down.

Once you fully appreciate that perspective, the world starts to occur to you as a lot less crazy and you can finally understand the secret they don't want you to know.

Of course, this is something you will never hear via the mainstream. Until you accept the possibility that the mainstream does not report the news, but *constructs* it, you will be stuck in its constant, mind-numbing cycle of insanity.

"No one is going to give you the education you need to overthrow them. Nobody is going to teach you your true history, teach you your true heroes, if they know that that knowledge will help set you free." ~ Assata Shakur

Yes, the illusion appears all-encompassing, but it *is* all illusion nonetheless. And the simple truth is this…

Bullshit only works *through our consent.*

The psychopaths have *never* wielded complete power and total, authoritarian control, except through deception. The only reason we believe they have ultimate power is because they have *caused us to believe they have ultimate power.*

Surely that is the core message from the 1939 movie *The Wizard of Oz*. Picture the Wizard, cowering behind his curtain, desperately trying to pull on levers and push buttons to maintain his crumbling illusion… and consider that that is exactly what the Owners are doing right now!

Of course they must be panicking. It is totally understandable when you realize their identity is fundamentally connected to their idea of being some kind of superior class—or even *race*—compared to the rest of us.

What's more, that giant, booming hologram does not tower over us because the Owners *hate* us, but because they *fear* us. Because they know the truth.

"You let one ant stand up to us, then they all might stand up. Those puny little ants outnumber us a hundred to one. And if they ever figure that out, there goes our way of life! It's not about food. It's about keeping those ants in line." ~ Hopper, A Bug's Life

We cannot be allowed to gain the knowledge that will set us free. Following the principles of propaganda, we have all been lied to from childhood, and the lies have been repeated so often that they appear true. That's why the revolutionary leader Malcolm X stated, "Only a fool would let his enemy teach his children."

Perhaps it is more accurate to say that we have not really been enslaved, but rather *bewitched* by a spell, chanted monotonously out of every media outlet.

"...the rank and file are usually much more primitive than we imagine. Propaganda must therefore always be essentially simple and repetitious." ~ Joseph Goebbels

The way propaganda works is just like the way that elephant trainers in Asia found they could control their animals. They start by tying one end of a rope round a baby elephant's leg and then fix the other end to a stake hammered into the ground. The baby elephant pulls and pulls but soon learns the stake is immovable. As the elephant grows into maturity, all it takes is a small peg driven into the ground and the enormous beast will not even attempt to escape, not because it is powerless, but because it *believes* it is powerless.

That is how bullshit works, through mass delusion. We believe we must obey only because we have been *taught to believe* we must obey.

The Owners had to invent so many layers of bullshit precisely *because* they are so few in number and therefore could never control us through overt force or violence alone.

"Appear weak when you are strong, and strong when you are weak." ~ Sun Tzu, The Art of War

The Owners created their elaborate web of illusion in order to appear strong despite the fact that they possess little real power. But in reality they are the Wizard, they are the elephant trainer. They are not strong, *we are strong*, we are the elephant!

They constructed the web of illusion by taking over the dominant social narrative, through *buying complete control* over all the channels that construct what we accept as reality, including politics, media, religion, lawmaking, education, and science, and also by outlawing dialog that might seek to explore alternative worldviews.

"Psychedelics are illegal not because a loving government is concerned that you may jump out of a third story window. Psychedelics are illegal because they dissolve opinion structures and culturally laid down models of behavior and information processing. They open you up to the possibility that everything you know is wrong." ~ Terence McKenna

It is only through the constant and universal tidal wave of bullshit that the Owners have gained their apparent dominance, and yet that could only have been achieved by persuading the masses to step up and accept our domination *voluntarily*.

The solution is stunningly simple. We only need to break out of the bullshit within the scope of our own minds.

See it for what it is, just bullshit. It is not inherently evil, and it is certainly not to be feared, no more than shadows flickering on the wall. As the sovereign master of your own mind, only you get to choose what you believe or disbelieve.

If our chains are no more than mental, then we can get free simply by changing our consciousness, as James Lindsay explained in his 2020 essay *Psychopathy and the Origins of Totalitarianism*.

"What, then, could possibly be the answer to this perilous and perennial tangle? Fortunately, the first step, at the least, is very simple. It's mere awareness. It is learning to recognize the constructed pseudo-reality for what it is—a fabricated simulation of reality that is unfit for human societies—and beginning to reject unapologetically any demand to participate in it...

In the exact instant one becomes competent at spotting the lie—or, the network of lies—held in service of a constructed pseudo-reality and its social enforcement, one already possesses the necessary perspective to break the spell of the pseudo-reality in its entirety...

The way resistance—just plain resistance—works is by restoring to the normal person the epistemic and moral authority necessary to resist the ideologue's illegitimate demands to participate in a pseudo-real fraud. That is, it restores confidence in normality to the normal. No one feels ashamed of resisting a con, whatever form it takes, and this is the real phenomenon we face with any growing ideological pseudo-reality. Its paralogic and paramorality work to drain us of our sense of authority to know what is and is not true and what is and is not right. One's authority only lacks under the assumptions of the paralogical and paramoral systems, however—that is, inside pseudo-reality— and it can be reclaimed by anyone who simply refuses to participate in the lie. Step outside of the pseudo-reality (take the "red pill," as depicted in The Matrix), and you'll see."

All we need to do is seek the truth and tell our truth, as it appears to us. Show that the Emperor is wearing no clothes. Pull back the curtain to reveal the Wizard and his manipulative machinations. When the pursuit of truth is encouraged, not dictated by Big Money that controls the mainstream narrative, each of us can be free to make up our own minds, wherever that may lead.

Above all, we can each reserve the right to say "yes" or to say "no", in particular when it concerns our body and mind, over which, as John Stuart Mill put so elegantly, "the individual is sovereign".

After taking back ownership, we will discover new opportunities to make changes in other areas of life. That is all that is needed. All it takes is enough of us. But first we have to break the conditioning that has been instilled in us our whole lives that unthinking obedience to the State is a moral obligation. It is not, as history has taught time and again. Rather, once we see clearly we are under a more profound moral obligation to resist. As James Lindsay wrote, "No one feels ashamed of resisting a con."

That little word "no" has enormous potential to create space that invites in new possibilities. Here is one way you may start to apply it judiciously in your own life. If we can offer one simple touchstone as a starting point for every individual to help bring about the nonviolent revolution the world needs now, it would have to be...

"Don't buy their shit."

We have *quite literally* bought into the lies. We have continually parted with our hard-earned money (which represents our time and energy, our very life force) to acquire shit we don't need, including their toxic food and their toxic propaganda.

We have been trained to give up the best years of our lives in return for nothing more than money to pump back into the global vending machine in order to get fed shit! That insane fundamental commercial exchange is the foundation of the whole System.

And, as soon as we see it for what it is, we get to choose. We can choose not to buy their shit any longer, and instead *reclaim* our sovereign authority and rediscover the essence of our ancestral humanity, piece by piece.

"The system will collapse, if we refuse to buy what they are selling — their ideas, their version of history, their wars, their weapons, their notions of inevitability. Remember this: We be many and they be few. They need us more than we need them. Another world is not only possible, she is on her way. On a quiet day, I can hear her breathing." ~ Arundhati Roy

If we no longer choose to participate in the System, all we need to do is simply smile and say "no", to choose not to buy their shit, whether it's the "food-like products" on the shelves or the narrow, divisive belief systems. We choose instead to celebrate freedom over health choices and over thought.

"The only way to deal with an unfree world is to become so absolutely free that your very existence is an act of rebellion." ~ Albert Camus

We do not even have to hate their System, parasitical and psychopathic and fake as it may be. If you or I decide that it does not work for us, no further justification is required. We may simply say the quiet and powerful counter-spell "No thanks."

Nobody knows exactly what will happen next, or what we must do, but it will involve saying, "No thank you". If and when enough of us say "No", it simply all ends and we get to start over.

Let us unpick some of the strands of the Owners' spell, so we may choose what we might keep, and what we may choose to decline.

One of the greatest imprisoning bullshit myths is how we have allowed the State to dictate morality. Let us be clear: that is neither the State's job nor its right!

Chief among the poisonous fruits of the false morality the Owners have sold us is how it has been allowed to pervert our desire to *care* for one another. In recent years our innate instinct to love our home and our tribe has been deliberately mutated into a global guilt trip.

Furthermore, lurking beneath that universal guilt, their New Original Sin, is an even more insidious and foul implication: that the appropriate response is to hate humanity itself! As the Club of Rome decreed in *The First Global Revolution (1991)*, "The common enemy of humanity is Man."

Under the spell of this black magic, the finger of blame is pointed against the whole of humanity, dividing us against each other, prompting anger toward our fellow human beings. Generation after generation we have been sold a pack of lies that have divided us into opposing groups based on race, religion, politics, and a plethora of other bullshit false dichotomies.

Their absurd premise is that, even though humanity was naturally able to dwell harmoniously in nature for almost the entirety of its existence, we somehow suddenly lost that ability within the space of a few centuries.

All the while, attention and blame have been deflected away from the true polluters. The implication is that, by being consumers of the global vending machine with its plastic products and shrink-wrapped food-like edibles, *we* are the ones who must carry the blame, including for the emergence of that intangible specter that is "climate change", surely not the trans-global corporations, which after all exist only to serve our insatiable greed.

Furthermore, the authoritarian System argues that, because humans are inherently violent and immoral, we obviously need to be controlled and policed. Of course, if you read the newspapers and watch the news, there is overwhelming evidence to support this version of reality. The world is a dangerous place because it is full of unstable, greedy, stupid people.

But is that true? Is that what you see when you look in the mirror? Is that what you experience with your own senses as you go about your day-to-day life? If you believe in kindness, forgiveness, cooperation, sharing, helping your neighbors, why would you think that is not intrinsic, universal human nature?

If you ignore the television and instead meet people face to face, you will realize the simple truth. Wherever you go, you find that the vast majority of people on Earth believe in love, kindness, and generosity, traits that are quite alien to the psychopath, but which they are nevertheless more than happy to pervert and to exploit.

Of course, when people live under a constant cloud of fear, they do manifest antisocial behaviors such as jealousy, greed, and violence. But that is not who we truly *are*.

Humanity is not the enemy. You are not our enemy, we are not yours. Perhaps whoever told us that we are our own enemy is the only enemy. *They* are the enemy of freedom; they are the enemy of any true, natural, thriving human society.

Ask yourself, is it in *our* interests to suffer under such widespread mistrust? How can it be? Or is it in *theirs*?

Their misanthropy dogma is not just limited to the climate change argument but consequently further fuelled by the vegan and animal rights movements, which now seem to be given free rein in the media. Within the span of a single generation, society seems to have decided that not only is the choice of an ancestral, animal-based diet chiefly responsible for destroying the environment, but also that it is now ethically indefensible.

But *why* are we now told that suddenly our biggest problems are global? The answer lies in that age-old mechanism that has been used for millennia to control the masses through bullshit: problem > reaction > solution.

Because our problems are now evidently global, the only possible solutions must by definition also be global, and that means our salvation can only come from above, in other words through some kind of New World Order.

Yet pay attention to the middle step: reaction. It is the Owners that served up the globalized problems, and they are also the ones offering a global solution as the only remedy. But first we have to react, and therein lies another key to refuting their magic spell.

Remember, bullshit only works with our consent! The spell has power only if *we* step up and demand to be rescued from ourselves! They need us to volunteer, to walk willingly into the slaughterhouse. Why? Because they cannot force us, because they do not hold the real power.

According to the case for humanity's prosecution, there is only one realistic solution. *We* must accept that our species is naturally bad, that we are not capable of discerning right from wrong for ourselves and of organizing our own society accordingly, that the world is a dangerous place, and ultimately *we* must insist on adopting their New World Order.

They cannot force it on us. It only works if we accept their bullshit and react accordingly. Why? Because we have the power! We always did. And, once we realize that, we discover we have the power to choose.

That means we also have the power to decide, according to the evidence of our senses and the still, small voice of truth in our own hearts, that humanity is not inherently evil, selfish, or immoral, and that maybe our woes stem from a tiny minority that is psychopathic.

Ask yourself if that whole belief system truly represents you and serves you. If not, if we have free will, perhaps we can choose another path, to say "no, thank you", to throw out their mythology of Original Sin and replace it with something different.

Perhaps, if we just change our own minds and choose to perceive the world differently, according to our truth, the world will in fact also transform.

"We but mirror the world. All the tendencies present in the outer world are to be found in the world of our body. If we could change ourselves, the tendencies in the world would also change. As a man changes his own nature, so does the attitude of the world change towards him. This is the divine mystery supreme. A wonderful thing it is and the source of our happiness. We need not wait to see what others do." ~ Mahatma Gandhi

The Owners know the eternal truth of this sentiment. We act out division, jealousy, discrimination, hatred because that is the picture that has been painted for us since childhood. All we need to do is repaint the mental picture.

We take responsibility. We confess that we were the ones who sleepwalked into this mess.

We also acknowledge that the Owners have been able to dominate us only because we chose to believe when we were told that the world was a hostile place; that we were victims who needed protection; that we deserved to be dominated!

We chose the comfort of not having to think for ourselves, of not having to be responsible for ourselves.

We admit that *we* stepped up and allowed ourselves to be divided and conquered. And that means that *we* can now choose something else, to be united and truly interdependent.

We bought your shit, and now we claim our sovereign right to make new choices.

One of our choices is to proclaim that division, hatred, and mistrust no longer serve our vision of humanity or of the world we choose to inhabit together.

We choose to say "no" to division and rivalries and instead to accept all others as the sovereign beings they were born to be.

We choose to celebrate not being sure, to explore and share ideas together, to honor our differences and the outliers who help us to contemplate new ideas.

We choose a world where love and respect rule, for no other reason than that is what we choose.

"They fear love because it creates a world they can't control."
~ George Orwell

Chapter 20:
Revolution Part Two: Your Health

"A wise man ought to realize that health is his most valuable possession." ~ Hippocrates

The System has done everything it can to hide the truth from you, so that it can continue to profit from your poor dietary education and eating habits, and then later again from your failing health.

"For the first fifty years of your life, the food industry is trying to make you fat. Then, the second fifty years, the pharmaceutical industry is treating you for everything." ~ Pierre Dukan

Fortunately, due to the nature of bullshit, *everything the System can do* is still not quite enough. Once you see through the bullshit and understand how it wants to entice you away from the way nature designed humans to live, you can easily break out of the System's spell and make simple alternative choices that work better for you.

"It's a big club, and you ain't in it. You and I are not in the big club. And by the way, it's the same big club they use to beat you over the head with all day long when they tell you *what to believe*." ~ George Carlin

Now that we have reclaimed our right to choose *what to believe for ourselves*, this chapter will set out steps you can take right now to reclaim your natural human vitality. Remember, the System does not want you to be healthy. Only *you* can reclaim your health.

Let us make it clear at this point that the authors do not presume to tell you what you should or should not eat. We respect and stand for your right as a sovereign individual to make your own choices, and we also believe strongly that those should be fully informed choices. In order to support that, our purpose with this chapter is to summarize the information we have covered so far in this book.

Also please be assured that you are far from alone at this crossroads where the long road of miseducation meets the path to freedom. There is a massive movement happening all around you right now; millions of people are rediscovering the benefits of a species-appropriate, high-fat, low-carbohydrate diet after several generations of deliberately health-destroying propaganda. But don't wait for confirmation from the mainstream that this movement exists before you choose to join it, because then it will certainly be too late.

"This is the new medicine, which is going to take thirty years to be accepted. But, as far as your health is concerned, you better accept it today, you haven't got thirty years to wait for medicine to catch up." ~ Professor Tim Noakes

The simplistic solution to the obesity epidemic that the System proposes is "eat less, move more", which will suck you into fad diets and relentless excess physical activity. Diets fail more than nine times out of ten, and frankly trying to exercise your way to your proper shape is just plain unnecessary.

That's because the root cause of obesity is not the oversimplified imbalance of "calories in versus calories out", but rather the modern fake food-like products that send your body all the wrong signals, keeping it locked in a kind of accelerated winter preparation fat-storage mode 365 days of the year. The plain reality is that, just as modern hunter-gatherer tribes do today, you too can achieve a healthy physical form by choosing to combine a way of eating that is consistent with your natural design with a moderate amount of physical activity.

As a bonus, taking back control over your nutrition will also mean you can avoid most of the factors that are behind the epidemics of chronic, non-communicable illnesses currently engulfing the modern world. Seven out of the eleven top causes of death in 2020, including heart disease, cancer, stroke, and diabetes, have their root in metabolic dysfunction, and that in turn comes straight from diet. It is no surprise that all these health crises hit the modern world at the same time as obesity suddenly became the norm.

While the general population is sadly resigned to the reality that chronic disease is now a normal part of human life, it is in fact an anomaly that should appall us. As outlier high-fat advocate Dr. Barry Groves explained,

"Civilized man is the planet's only chronically sick animal. No wild animal or human culture living on its natural diet suffers the chronic diseases we do."

Groves adds as a footnote that the only other species that are affected happen to be our domestic pets, who suffer many of the same diseases as we do, and for the exact same reasons!

"Why must we accept as normal what we find in a race of sick and weakened human beings?" ~ Dr. Herbert M. Shelton

With open eyes, the appropriate rational responses to witnessing the unfolding collapse in health of the world's population ought to be astonishment and outrage. We should not shy away from those emotions, but rather use them to channel our energies in positive directions.

Do we consent to being swept along with this trend, to standing in silence as we witness not only the inevitable slide towards sickness and death of those around us, but of our entire civilization as well? Do we have another choice besides sacrificing all that is good and wholesome at the altar of corporate profits and gross domestic product?

Fortunately there is also good news, which is that we *can* rediscover our natural state of healthfulness! If the night is darkest before the dawn, as the psalm says, then surely we could be on the verge of a new dawn for the human race, our era of regeneration.

If, as we have seen clearly documented, mice and rats and cats and humans can *degenerate* within the span of even a single generation, why should we not also have the potential to *regenerate* our bodies just as rapidly?

If our core genetics must be unchanged, surely all we need is to restore appropriate nutrition, giving our bodies everything they need and less of what they don't, and to rediscover healthy lifestyles that put us back in our proper place among nature's cycles.

Perhaps we can become free-range humans once again. Obviously that does not mean winding the clock back several thousand years and returning to the old hunter-gatherer lifestyles that support only one human being per square mile of land. No, times have changed, and instead we now have the opportunity to get creative and build something new out of the rubble of the old System!

Clearly, reclaiming our true sovereignty and self-determination over our own health requires we change deeply ingrained habits, and that necessitates a shift in thinking. So let's now summarize the journey we have taken through this book and redefine what we think of as "food".

Our bodies and brains need both fuel and nourishment. The many observations of nature and human history that we have explored through previous chapters provide conclusive evidence that the majority of what is being presented as "food" today—now constituting an astonishing seventy percent of the "standard American diet"—*just isn't*!

In fact, if we trace the human devolution timeline, what we think of as "food" actually falls into three simple, quite distinct categories:

- **Ancestral foods** cover anything that a Paleolithic ancestor who lived in your part of the world fifty thousand years ago would recognize and know how to use. That means sources of sustenance derived directly from nature, which could very likely be preserved with minimal manual processing.

- **Traditional foods** are those that entered our diet within the last few thousand years following the end of the last Ice Age and the advent of the worldwide Agricultural Revolution. These include all varieties of domesticated fruits, vegetables and grains that have existed for hundreds of years, together with a few more highly processed ingredients like sugar and spices. Think of any foodstuffs that your great-great-grandma would recognize and know how to use.

- Finally, we have the **industrial era's "food-like products"**, all invented in the past few generations, which we have already established are responsible for the explosion in obesity and the majority of chronic disease.

If we work on the principle that "food" is that which both nourishes and satisfies, evidently only the first two categories can be considered "food"! Let's now review and understand the three types in more detail.

First, **ancestral food**: anything you know that a caveman or cavewoman would recognize. If you were to show them a modern breed of cow, hog, or deer any one of them would know (better than practically anyone alive today) *exactly* what to do with it, and how to carry out the minimal processing required to eat it now or to preserve it to be eaten in the near future, in addition to making countless other creative and useful products from what was left over.

As previously mentioned, wherever else you look in nature, all animals eat the food that *that type of animal eats*. All lions eat warm-blooded herbivores; all orcas eat seals; all gorillas eat leafy plants; all koalas eat eucalyptus leaves… and they always have done. So we can state with certainty the obvious fact that the appropriate diet for any species of animal is *the food that species has always eaten*.

Ancestral foods are those natural sources of nourishment *that human beings have always eaten*. Therefore ancestral food is our most natural, species-appropriate, and—by extension— healthiest source of nourishment. They include: the meat, fat, bone marrow, and offal from large animals; eggs and honey when available; a wide range of smaller game animals; fish and shellfish; plus seasonal wild nuts, fruits, and berries; certain mosses and fungi; together with a few edible wild plants if the preferred foods were not available.

Our caveman ancestors will certainly have employed a range of basic processes to help keep food edible for longer, such as the use of fire, cold, and salt. Preservation will have been extremely important, not only because it meant less work was needed to get enough to eat and ensuring they had a supply through lean periods, but also helping to minimize humanity's impact on the environment.

We can therefore state that *all of these foods* are species-appropriate for humans, when obtained from the local ecosystem at the relevant time of year. They comprise the most nutritious and complete diet we can have, and we know they will give us what our bodies need and very little that they don't. We can also infer that they put the least strain on our systems, because our bodies instinctively recognize them thanks to countless years of adaptation.

"Is mother nature a psychopath? Why would she design foods to shorten the lifespan of the human race?" ~ Joanna Blythman

We can know these things as true from the fact that our ancestors not only survived but thrived to become the most widespread species on Earth. Of course, in biological terms, with the exception of some recent loss of physical stature and brain size, we modern humans are still pretty much identical to our Paleolithic forebears.

The bottom line: You can eat whatever true, ancestral food you like and put minimal stress on the body.

Now we move on to **traditional food**. This encompasses any novel foodstuffs from the Pliocene era, spanning the period from the start of the Neolithic through the Agricultural Revolution up to pre-industrial times just a few centuries ago. Traditional foodstuffs include all domesticated fruits, vegetables, and nuts together with some more recent processed items like refined sugar, orange juice, and whole wheat flour. In short, anything a Paleolithic ancestor may not recognize, but that you could expect to find in great-great-grandma's kitchen.

This era of human food history also introduced further methods of artisan processing, still firmly rooted in the need for preservation, such as pickling, fermenting, and canning.

As we have seen from the evidence, when consumed in excess this class of nutrient-poor, agricultural-era food can clearly put *some* stress on the human body, contributing to dis-ease, obesity, and other problems, as many farming cultures discovered to their cost. However, it is surely possible to source complete nutrition with a combination of ancestrally-appropriate and agricultural food sources, as most people still did just a few generations ago.

The bottom line: As they contain more starch, more sugar, and more plant anti-nutrients, traditional (non-ancestral) foodstuffs will put some stress on the body. However, your body is good at tolerating some stress, which is why we suffered very little obesity and chronic disease prior to the twentieth century. Unless you are already sick, you will probably get away just fine with eating some traditional food alongside the most nutrient-dense ancestral food.

Finally, we get to **not-food-at-all industrial food-like facsimiles**.

While this third category contains much of what people today think of as "food", it is patently nothing of the sort, because it fails the basic tests of *nourishing and satisfying the human being*.

A problem with many modern plant-derived foods is that they have been progressively bred and hybridized to enhance only those factors that serve the market's need for profit such as yield and a standardized appearance… but not for nutritional value!

Other modern processes, from the application of pesticides and herbicides to our fields as well as the addition of artificial preservatives, sweeteners, and flavor enhancers, only serve further to promote the interests of profits over the health of the people and the land.

The net result is the plethora of industrial, ultra-processed "human fodder", cheap, mass-produced ingredients reconstituted into shapes, textures, and colors designed to resemble food that are pumped out of factories day after day. As we have seen, most of the products of the modern food System are derived from row crops that are almost devoid of nutrients, anti-nutritious or even positively toxic.

The bottom line: Industrial food is so high in antinutrients and toxins, and so low in nutritional value, that it overwhelms the body's ability to deal with stress, and therefore has directly caused the explosions in obesity and chronic disease.

Let us now offer a few simple tests you can use to help distinguish real food from fake. If you only had to remember one, the handiest rule-of-thumb is probably this…

"Food commonly eaten for more than 150 years should be innocent until proven guilty, and food invented in the last 150 years is guilty until proven innocent." ~ Miles Hassell, MD

Applying that principle, as they are also very recent inventions, any novel genetically-modified (GMO) produce should also go into this category.

Here are some other useful questions to ask…

Where was it made?

Real food has always been made around the campfire or in a kitchen, never in a factory. If it is the product of an industrial plant, it isn't food! Food is natural, seasonal, satisfying, and naturally delivers balanced nutrition.

Who made it?

Was it made by machines or by human beings? Would it be possible to find out who grew or raised it and who prepared it for you, or is it the product of a vast, untraceable, unknowable, faceless, soulless chain of production and logistics processes?

Why was it made?

Was the motive purely profit, or was it crafted with love and skill in order to deliver true pleasure and vitality? Did somebody take the time and care to make it the best it could be?

What's it made of?

Counting ingredients is a far more helpful indicator of healthfulness than counting calories. A long list of ingredients is usually a clear sign of fake, ultra-processed products. Looking at the ingredients, could you confidently identify *where in nature* you might go to find every one? Did each one once roam or grow or be sourced from the land or sea? (Good luck finding a natural source of soy lecithin or pea protein isolate.)

Where did it come from?

Humans have always thrived on what their immediate environment offered, therefore our natural way of eating is local and seasonal. Did all the ingredients originate somewhere around your local area? Do you have any idea where they came from, or when they were sourced?

Does it all look the same?

Any examples of naturally-sourced food will always come with a variety of inconsistent appearance. Fake alternatives produced by machines in factories always feature the exact same characteristics.

Could you make it in a kitchen?

You should be able to recreate any real food in a regular kitchen, given basic equipment and the appropriate skills. If it can only be made in an industrial laboratory, it isn't food.

Will anything else consume it?

If you leave margarine outside, for example, not even ants and slugs will touch it. Many ultra-processed products are packed with so many preservatives that not even bacteria can digest them. They can literally look unchanged after years! Feel free to test this for yourself.

Does it bring joy?

Real food that has been prepared with love is one of our most fundamental sources of pleasure, leaving you satiated, satisfied, and happy. Food-like products may deliver a short-term flavor hit or a rush from sugar and caffeine, but that is often followed by a comedown, and the overall effect is not to create lasting happiness.

Does it satisfy?

Another telling sign of faked foods is how, like drugs, they can leave you craving another hit very soon afterwards. On the other hand, if your body recognizes that it is properly nourished, you will naturally not feel the desire to keep eating. You don't get that with food-like products, which are designed to maximize consumption in the name of profit.

Is it cheap?

We have been groomed to expect, and even demand, cheap sustenance as though it is a human right. But consider that perhaps the food we eat, if it properly nourishes, satisfies, delivers health and brings joy, if it has had the proper time and love invested into raising and preparing it… should not be cheap! Perhaps we should all be looking to spend more on our food in return. However, note that when you do choose to invest in highly nutritious food sources you will need much less of it, so it may not end up costing any more!

Instead of seeking what is most affordable, we will do much better to choose what to eat based on nutritional density. Remember, the modern world is fat and yet still hungry *not* because we are overfed but because we are *under-nourished*!

Ultra-processed food-like products not only fail to nourish our bodies, but in fact are expressly designed *not* to satisfy our appetites! If you get enough nutrition, you can be healthy and vibrant, and you simply will not want to keep eating.

Ultimately, surely the best thing you can do is to try it *for yourself*. Your body knows, so listen to it. However, remember that modern fake food is highly addictive by design, so be kind to yourself and give your body time to adjust as it gets over the changes, particularly the powerful cravings that sugar and wheat produce. You will very likely have massive colonies of carb-addicted bacteria in your digestive system, which actually release chemicals that mimic hunger hormones as they die off, and it takes time to ride that out.

It is easy to monitor your own state of health... How well do you sleep? How refreshed and recharged do you feel when you wake in the morning? What signals do you get from how your guts feel? How are your teeth, your hair quality, your joints, your sex drive, et cetera?

It was never the job of the Government to look after our health. For ninety-nine percent of our existence, we managed just fine without scientists to tell us what we should or shouldn't put in our mouths.

Now we can use our journey back to real, natural food to rediscover our own *lore*. When, individually and together, we figure out for ourselves, over time, what works for us, we too can thrive again, as Weston Price wrote in *Nutrition and Physical Degeneration*.

"In my studies of these several racial stocks I find that it is not accident but accumulated wisdom regarding foods that lies behind their physical excellence and freedom from our modern degenerative processes, and, further, that on various sides of our world the primitive people know many of the things that are essential for life-things that our modern civilizations apparently do not know. These are the fundamental truths of life that have put them in harmony with Nature through obeying her nutritional laws. Whence this wisdom? Was there in the distant past a world civilization that was better attuned to Nature's laws and have these remnants retained that knowledge? If this is not the explanation, it must be that these various primitive racial stocks have been able, through a superior skill in interpreting cause and effect, to determine for themselves what foods in their environment are best for producing human bodies with a maximum of physical fitness and resistance to degeneration."

In addition to what we eat, we should surely also take time to apply a similar line of questioning to *how we eat*.

Clearly our ancestral lifestyle was starkly different to the way we live today with recent concepts such as microwaved TV dinners, snacks on the go, and drive-throughs. Today we are not only eating far more and far more frequently, but thinking about our food far less. Often we even eat entirely unconsciously, barely noticing what we have stuffed into our mouths.

You will very likely find that, when your body realizes it is properly nourished, you will not feel the urge to eat three times a day, plus snacking between meals. To quote Zoë Harcombe, "Unless you are a cow, or you want to be the size of one, please stop grazing!" With proper food, some days you may not even bother to eat at all, which is very likely in tune with the ancestral pattern.

Using good, calorie-dense animal fat as fuel is like burning coal on a fire, it burns hot and long, whereas living on mainly carbs is like trying to feed your fire with newspaper.

Just like how babies cry when they are hungry, many of us in the modern world have never grown out of that infantile relationship with food. That is unsurprising if the sustenance you're getting never actually satisfies, leaving your body constantly craving. Give your body the nutrition it needs and you will also discover that the discomfort, even the fear, of being hungry diminishes.

A further issue is that many of us, females in particular, are raised to equate the act of feeding our families with expressing love. That is totally natural. But again, when the food is fake and toxic, even that most basic of human loving acts is perverted into an unwitting form of abuse.

It is not only our bodies that are suffering in the modern day, but also our minds, spirits, relationships, and social bonds. Could restoring food to its natural place in our daily lives also help us to regenerate emotionally, and even help regenerate our families and communities?

Human life was always intimately tied to sourcing and sharing food. Food was our connection to nature and to each other. But the System had to separate us from our own nature and from the natural world so that we would become dependent on it for our existence.

Today the communal role of food has been stripped away and replaced with the false blessing we call convenience. As we have seen, that has come at a great price, which is the loss of an essential part of our humanity, our connection to our tribe and to our ancestors through a shared way of life. That is the great atrocity.

Let's not forget that the very earliest form of recorded history is cave paintings, and what did our ancestors choose to depict? They painted what was *most important* in their lives: scenes of animals and hunting.

Surely today we have no less need for significance and purpose, which comes from seeing and enjoying the results of our labor. The modern abstraction of working in order to get money to be able to meet our basic needs via products and services provided by various third parties has stripped that purpose away from us.

Ever since then, throughout all recorded history, people have asked why we are here. Perhaps the answers are very simple.

"Let us go to the ignorant savage, consider his way of eating, and be wise." ~ Professor Ernest Hooten, *Apes, Men, and Morons*

But, short of all running out into the wilderness with spears, how else can we use food to get closer to our true, ancestral relationship with other humans and with nature?

Clearly, now that practically all the land is owned, we cannot all hope to be self-sufficient. But we can still find creative ways to regenerate our relationship with food: how we source it, prepare it, enjoy it, and give thanks for it.

There are good reasons why we are still biologically and emotionally drawn to our natural, direct, highly involved relationship with food. That is why, despite the distraction of convenience, so many of us still love to hunt, fish, garden, cook and bake, to stand at the barbecue or stare into the campfire…

Those activities are embedded deep in our instincts, they connect us to our natural birthright, because food has always represented more than energy, but the very flow of life's natural forces.

Consider how every animal is born with the genetic knowledge of how to be that kind of animal. For example, if you take ex-battery hens, who have never seen the sun before and have only ever been fed grain through a tube, release them free-range and they will immediately get busy scratching for bugs and worms in the leaf litter.

If other animals have those innate instincts, surely it makes sense that humans are born *knowing* how to be humans. That's why we don't need to be told to enjoy being outdoors, sitting around a fire, or finding our own food!

Instead of exclusively going out to work to earn money so that you can put food on the table, can you invest some of your time more creatively? Consider how you can source good food that is local, natural, and seasonal. How can you shorten—or eliminate—the supply chain, perhaps by visiting farmers' markets or building direct relationships with local producers?

Your spending power can make a small but significant difference. How can you use your money to support those sources of food that matter most to you? This revolution is not a call to arms, but *a call to farms*!

Time is our most precious resource. In many ways, how we give our time represents what we value and love most, so *give your food your time*.

Take time to source and prepare the best ingredients, learning and sharing new skills along the way.

Wherever you go in the world, sharing food is a universal way of honoring both friends and strangers. Take time to sit down with your loved ones to enjoy what you have prepared together.

All traditional cultures have a practice of giving thanks for food. Today that is very much the exception, so shouldn't we put it back? (Some scientists now believe that appreciating food and water could even change it on an atomic level!)

Instead of always rushing onto the next thing, after enjoying a shared meal, take time to rest and digest. Let's make digestion trendy again!

These small changes may help us to regenerate not only our physical health, but also our relationships with ourselves and with each other. What's more, they may help us remember what it means to be human.

Picture a thousand ancestors who are no longer here physically, but whom you may remember in spirit. See their faces smiling back kindly at you, their nods of approval as you sit down with your loved ones, the latest generation of humans once more choosing to share what really matters.

Also imagine the grief and horror they might feel at the realization that the modern, perverted equivalent of our tribal leaders are plotting to take that right away from us.

Chapter 21:
Revolution Part Three:
Society

We started to contemplate the necessary revolution with the essential first step of taking back control over our minds, reclaiming our own individual right to choose what to believe. In the second part we looked at how we may reclaim our health by telling the truth about the three different classes of "food".

In this final chapter we will show why having the information to make informed food choices is ultimately futile unless we also have the freedom to act on those choices. If society decides to prohibit our ancestral, species-appropriate diet then we will no longer be free to choose it. That is why we will now complete our journey by presenting the case for a necessary food revolution as, and on behalf of, the entire human race, and why we believe that food sovereignty must be where humanity draws the line.

It is often said about food that "you are what you eat," but the eternal truth in this simple statement applies at a far more profound level than basic health. Just as the proper ordained place of every living being within the web of life is defined by what it consumes and what it is consumed by, food represents in a very real sense *who we are*.

We can also see how food is an inseparable requirement for living a fulfilled human life. In 1943, Abraham Maslow proposed that individuals are motivated by a set of universal imperatives that he arranged in a logical progression, building up from the most basic *biological* needs, through *safety, belonging, esteem,* and ultimately *self-actualization*.

Looking at the way humans always lived prior to agriculture, it is easy to imagine how the way that life revolved around the search for food would have played an important role in achieving every one of the stages in Maslow's model.

Beyond meeting just our basic *physiological* needs through providing our nutritional and energy requirements, the confidence that we have the capacity to provide enough sustenance to support ourselves and our loved ones is surely an important factor in our basic *security*. Imagine the feeling of confidence to know that your family could always feed itself no matter what life threw your way!

As we have already explored, throughout our existence, food must also have played a central role in our sense of *belonging*. Ancestral cultures would have been bonded together in the everyday communal quest for sustenance, through carefully observing the world around them, hunting and gathering, processing, preparing, sharing, and giving thanks for their food. It was the way we fundamentally both perceived and manifested our place in creation, through an intimate understanding of our environment, the passage of the seasons, and the movements of the heavens.

The sourcing of food surely also helped us to meet our need for *esteem*, by providing a regular feeling of accomplishment, because individuals' value to their tribe was linked not only to their ability to support each other but also to being part of the vitality and joy that gave.

In Maslow's Hierarchy of Needs, the highest level of achievement, *self-actualization,* is linked to realizing our creative potential. Surely that would have been given limitless scope for expression through solving the everyday problems presented by providing for our own needs and the needs of our tribe, responding to seasonal and environmental changes, and in gaining and sharing new skills.

Every day would have brought fresh new challenges and opportunities for development, which might involve creating shelter, designing tools, weapons and traps, coming up with hunting strategies, learning about animals, fungi, and herbs, or finding ways to make use of all the by-products from hunts.

From these understandings we can see how the central place of food in life was inseparable from not only what it always meant to be human, but also to be a fulfilled, happy human. Inseparable, that is, until the dawn of agriculture.

Consider how much we have lost since we gave up all that rich existence and handed the control of our daily lives over to others, eventually substituting it with what we have now, the endless pursuit of wages stretching over half a century of long, repetitive working weeks. By removing our ability to meet our own needs directly from the world around us, the System has robbed us of most of our natural sources of fulfillment and replaced them with infantile dependency.

The inevitable outcomes of that dependency on the System are plain to see: the degeneration of the human condition on every level!

Ever since the invention of land ownership and wealth, distracting and disassociating us from our true place in the natural order has been the essential foundation of the System's mechanisms of control. We have paid a very great price for that abomination against nature, and so has our beautiful Earth.

From what we now know, two vitally important conclusions become apparent, which together light the path to our remedy, how we can—and will—regenerate.

The first is that *we* have allowed ourselves to become divorced from nature through the process of being disconnected from our natural food, and that came at an enormous cost. It cost us our health, our sanity, and our true sense of community.

The second insight, as we have already discussed at some length, is that it was only achieved by means of extensive bullshit: they had to get us to step forward into servitude *willingly*.

Why did we go along with it? We complied because we are basically good and loving people who value peace and cooperation. While those same motives of course do not apply to the psychopaths in charge, who seek to dominate and to extract as much as they can for themselves, they have always relied on the fact that it *does* apply to the vast majority of us. They used it to disguise servitude to them and their System as cooperation for the good of "society", for the apparent benefit of all.

We also went along with it because they implied it was our obligation, when it is not. They led us to believe, quite falsely, that compliance is the righteous and virtuous path, and for a very important reason, which is because *they needed us to comply of our own accord.* That is why they had to use so many layers of bullshit to cover every angle and create an all-encompassing illusion... media propaganda, social pressure, programmed education, false science, and even religion, all to fool us into believing what is not real, coercing us into voluntary submission.

And it is still all only really held together by bullshit, and therefore it depends on our compliance. Most people are not even aware that the majority of what we perceive as immutable "laws" are not in fact laws at all, only *statutes*, and statutes are by definition *contractual*. In other words, we are only bound to comply with them by consent!

According to ancient and unvarying Common Law, the Owners could never *lawfully* enforce any man-made statute if doing so would violate our liberty, never mind those that violate human rights on a colossal scale... *against our consent*! They could only achieve it, and maintain order, by building and maintaining the mass illusion and manipulating the appearance of general consent.

We might wonder, if Common Law supersedes the Owners' Statute Law, is there perhaps some way we could pursue emancipation through the courts? History teaches that to wait for such an outcome would be a fool's hope, because the legal system must ultimately serve the interests of the most powerful. The System will never police itself voluntarily.

However, a study of recent social history also shows that there *have* been numerous concrete movements toward freedom, that they have *always* originated with the ordinary people, from *us*, and in every instance starting with expressions of resistance. In every one of these true social advances, small-scale disobedience growing into mass disobedience has invariably preceded any subsequent change in Law.

For example, the Civil Rights Movement may not have happened when it did without Rosa Parks' protest on the bus; the emancipation of India and other colonies only came about after massive popular rebellions; the end of slavery in the West was triggered by the Haitian Revolution. History books may focus on prominent men like Martin Luther King, Gandhi, and William Wilberforce, but the real change was always ignited when ordinary people stood up and disobeyed.

It was sledge hammers and pickaxes that brought down the Berlin Wall, not a lawmaker's pen. Perhaps we are now looking towards another Berlin Wall event, only this time on an even bigger scale.

Of course there have also been many examples of rebellions that were suppressed through the acute application of extreme violence. As George Orwell wrote, "All tyrannies rule through fraud and force, but once the fraud is exposed they must rely exclusively on force." That is how the System works, but turning on its own people is its last resort, and even that is doomed to fail when enough of the People stand up together.

Once again, we stress that this modern-day tyranny ultimately depends completely on compliance. When enough of us refuse to comply with it, *the System must comply with us*. Is the picture becoming clearer?

And we are now being directed to invoke the final stage of the spell, which will be voluntarily to surrender total control over our lives to a new world government that seeks to control everything, including our money, freedom of movement, and even the food we eat.

It will do no good to reclaim our personal food choices in the face of such a universal, totalitarian power grab. This is their final play, and this time what is at stake is *everything*!

And, while it may seem trivial, the fact that they are coming after our food really must be the final straw.

Just take a few moments really to contemplate the utter absurdity of the idea that anyone else should have the right to dictate what we can and cannot put into our own mouths.

It is beyond absurd, it is truly obscene. Our rights are innate, not bestowed by our public servants in government, and certainly not by unelected non-governmental organizations. The only proper role of government is to *protect and to defend our rights*, never to dictate or limit them! But we have been led to believe that we only enjoy whatever rights we still possess only on license from our leaders.

That degree of control in dictating another human being's food is only appropriate when dealing with infants, and that tells you all you need to know about how the System views us, as well as the extent to which it has molded us. In the System's worldview, all of the rest of us 99.99% are consumers, stock units, less than human.

What do we call it when people confine a living thing, prevent it from being able to pursue its natural instincts, and force it to consume cheap food in the interests of maximizing profit in place of health? We already have a term that fits perfectly: *factory farming*. While the vast majority of right-thinking people would agree that factory farming is an abomination when it is inflicted on cattle and pigs and chickens, surely it also perfectly describes what the System is doing *to us*!

Don't expect the System ever to acknowledge the fact of that great atrocity. By now you should realize it is futile to expect the mainstream to tell you the truth about anything! (Based on its track record, you are more likely to be better off believing and doing the opposite of whatever it tells you.)

The World Economic Forum and its partners in crime would have us believe that salvation will only come through a combination of even more technology and even more government. Yet countless generations thrived throughout human prehistory without those things, *and* their introduction has always coincided with, or precipitated, a sudden and catastrophic decline of humanity on every level, particularly in the last few centuries since the Industrial Revolution and the rise of the corporations and globalization. If politics is part of the problem, there can be no political solution. No, more technology and government cannot possibly be the solution we need.

The right to make *our own* decisions is absolutely fundamental and non-negotiable. The version of representative democracy we have today is all part of the bullshit, giving *the appearance* of self-determination through representation, when in reality our decision making has been abstracted out of our hands and given over to the minority who have the most money and influence.

As long as we continue to equate human civilization with rules and technological progress, we are doomed. Forget civilization, that does not need saving, at least in its current form. *The People do!*

When in tune with nature, the human body and mind possess incredible inherent capacities for healing dis-ease and restoring harmony. Surely human society must also possess a similar ability to heal itself. If so, our only path is clear, it requires that we find ways to move forward living in accordance *with* nature's laws instead of against them.

That is why, at this critical moment, food sovereignty is so vitally important. You might reclaim your own personal health—for now—but today the war against meat is already a hard reality, being waged all around us right now. It is no secret, widely broadcast on all channels across the public domain, and it constitutes nothing less than an assault on our freedom and our humanity.

And they are not even talking about presenting *alternative* choices; in their own words their ultimate goal is to eliminate your freedom to choose.

"Beef and lamb [to be] phased out by 2050 and replaced by greatly expanded demand for vegetarian food." ~ *Absolute Zero* report published by the University of Cambridge

The issue is not about anyone dictating to anyone else what is healthy or unhealthy. Ultimately, this revolution fights for our *right to choose* our own health path, and crucially to preserve that same right for our children and their children.

You should be free to make whatever dietary choices you like today or tomorrow, you may choose to eat a wholly plant-based diet… yet one day you may need meat, the most nutrient-dense, health-giving food available. Should you not then also have the right to make an alternative choice? And surely no sensible parent would wish to deny future generations from being free to make whatever choices may be right for them.

While we must of course reclaim the right to decide for ourselves what to eat, the grim reality remains that reclaiming personal sovereignty over our own health choices stands for nothing if Big Society is permitted to continue to dictate what is good for us.

"You'll eat much less meat… For the good of the environment and our health." ~ The World Economic Forum

Right now, many countries have their healthy eating guidelines, which of course are sponsored by Big Agriculture and the fake food-like product industry, and *today* we are still at liberty to ignore that guidance and to go about our lives as we see fit.

But the System is not stopping at advice. There are countless clear signs that the Owners ultimately intend to enforce the universal shift over to fake food.

"I do think all rich countries should move to 100% synthetic beef." ~ Bill Gates

They can achieve that shift through various means, all of which you can see playing out today. One tool at their disposal is to announce pandemics, outbreaks of invisible diseases like avian flu, that they will say necessitate the culling of entire flocks or herds of animals.

Another is a long-term strategy to apply pressure or to offer incentives to persuade animal farmers to turn their land over to crops or to woodland. We are already seeing this type of legislation on many fronts, including in the Netherlands, and the ridiculous Petition 13 presented by the State of Oregon, which would have required livestock to be allowed to live to a State-defined minimum age before slaughter and even sought to redefine artificial insemination as sexual abuse!

Finally, at the level of us, the consumers and taxpayers, they can exert ultimate control through systems of *digital social credit*. At the time of writing, a proposal for something called "Central Bank Digital Currency" is on the table at the G7 group of industrialized nations, and it includes one particularly terrifying adjective: "programmable".

"Programmable" means that this completely new form of "money" would not only be distributed by central banks (all of which are privately owned corporations not even answerable to democratically-elected governments), but that it could also be used to specify what types of transactions are permitted, *and which are prohibited*, on an individual basis.

Imagine a time in the very near future where it is not just corporations or countries that have emissions targets, but every one of us individually. That means that if some unelected NGO like the United Nations decides to decree that beef or lamb is so harmful that its supply must be strictly rationed, you will only be allowed to purchase a maximum amount each month.

Once cash is gone and the flow of money is all digital and programmable, should you attempt to purchase more of anything than the System deems appropriate, whether it is from a large store or from your local rancher, you may find your transaction blocked.

In other words, your food choices will *no longer be yours* to make. Instead you could find yourself forced to choose between buying soybeans, some lab-grown frankenmeat, or even bugs... or to starve!

That is the seriousness of the threat that faces us right now. If we give up these rights, we may find they are gone forever. That is why it is no exaggeration to say that this point in history could be humanity's last stand. Let food be where we, the People, draw the line!

If we are only left with the choice to support something that is fundamentally unlawful, trampling over our remaining rights and freedoms, or to rebel, rebellion is the only way to go. In taking that path we can be sure that we have right on our side.

"You may be the last generation which has the possibility to rebel. And if you don't rebel, there may be no more chances: humanity can be reduced to a robot-like existence. So rebel while there is still time!" ~ Osho

So what must we do? What form must our revolution take?

To retain our sovereign freedom to choose requires that, one way or another, we take back *our* society and prevent the Owners from ever again being able to dominate us, poison our minds, poison our bodies, or poison us against each other. Revolution is now our only option, not just at the individual level, but together as a united, sovereign human race.

If we are to reclaim our right to self-determination as a society, ultimately that means *the System has to go!* It is already too corrupt, with far too many layers of obfuscation between the real decision makers and the People who suffer the consequences. The psychopaths must be stopped and the whole thing taken down and built back better... but this time truly for the good of all.

"If we wait for the governments, it'll be too little, too late; if we act as individuals, it'll be too little; but if we act as communities, it might just be enough, just in time." ~ Rob Hopkins

Any one of us alone can do very little against the global System. It is only by reuniting and working together that we stand any chance.

Yes, it is true that they don't fear you... but they do fear *us*! You are not a threat to them... but *we* are.

If we stand together, acknowledging all our different lifestyles and beliefs, abandoning the false divisions that have kept us apart for too long, we *are* powerful. In fact, we must now stand together, because anything else would be suicidal. If we passively allow things to continue as they are, it is guaranteed that we will sacrifice not only our health, our own lives, but also that of the earth that sustains us, the very source of life.

We must find ways to move forward that serve humankind and our true place in the natural order, period.

And always remember, you are not alone! Of course they will try to make you think you are, which is why it is so important to connect with others. They may not be much like you, they may make different choices to yours, but freedom is about respecting each individual's right to make their own choices.

We are the 99.99%. *You* are the 99.99%!

Let us be clear, we do not need a violent revolution. When we realize that the power is *already* in our hands, even the idea of violence becomes redundant.

"Darkness cannot drive out darkness; only light can do that. Hate cannot drive out hate; only love can do that." ~ Martin Luther King, Jr.

Surely it is unnecessary to take back control over our lives by force, once we accept the truth that we have always had the control but have merely been tricked into believing that we did not.

Remember, the role of government is to *serve* us not to *rule* us! We are only ruled as long as we believe we are.

While politics is mainly a stage show, remember that bullshit is never all-encompassing, we don't live in a totalitarian state... quite yet! There are gaps in the bullshit, but if we fail to act now, those gaps will close and be gone forever.

The final spell they are trying to cast over us is to get *us* to demand *their* New World Order! Problem > Reaction > Solution!

It depends on us all *reacting* the way they're telling us we must, because that is presented as the only choice.

The world's current population finds itself in a situation that is unique in all of history. For the first time the problems presented to us through the media are global. The threat we face is now coming on all fronts, which is why we must all take a stand together.

If they can make the *problems* global, that justifies a global *solution*, which is of course the New World Order. But it is still just a spell, they cannot force it on us, because they do not have the power... they have to make us demand their rule, like the mythological vampire who only has power once invited into your home.

We must decline the Owners' offer of a new world government, instead declaring that we can fix our own problems locally, or at least that we should have the right to *try*. Who knows what could be possible if we direct our immense creativity into building a new way of living on Earth!

People, the true power is ours!

Seriously, using the evidence of our senses, can we actually *know* that we face real, tangible, global problems? If we cannot be completely sure then maybe the only global problem we really have is the globalists!

All that is needed is for enough people to say "No, thanks" to the New World Order and its global "solutions".

Remember, they need *us* to beg *them* for their help. And we are not going to. Instead we will stand shoulder to shoulder and declare, "No. We are not buying your shit, thanks, but we'll take our chances together. You've had millennia, you failed, now it's the People's turn."

So let's spread the word, and the word is "No."

"And then the people said 'no.' The end." ~ Anonymous Internet meme

It really is that simple.

Our future cannot be a new style of top-down organization of society. The next chapter for humanity will be rebuilt locally, quite literally from the grass roots!

It is already happening. More and more free-thinking individuals are choosing to reject the globalists' food-like substitutes, to reject dependency, to retire the plows and the giant agricultural machines and once again choosing sustainable ways of living built around real food and real community.

Instead of a worldwide supply chain, *we choose to* support our local ranchers who raise their animals naturally on rich, perennial pasture. We choose to regenerate the soil, and in the process we will regenerate our bodies, minds, and spirits as well as our communities.

It really is all connected, it is all the same web of life, and it all comes down to a simple choice: Nature's way or Man's.

Of course they will say we can't feed ourselves in a regenerative way. They will wave charts that show how only modern, industrial agriculture can feed the world. But that is not true. Apart from anything else, if you cannot feed people in a way that is sustainable in the long term, any further claim is automatically invalid.

"Agriculture doesn't cure famine, it promotes famine - it creates the conditions in which famines occur. Agriculture makes it possible for more people to live in an area than that area can support - and that's exactly where famines occur." ~ Daniel Quinn

The bottom line is, of course humanity *can* survive... but only if it is in line with nature's laws.

We must regenerate the soil because soil health drives plant health, which drives animal health, which drives our health.

If you subscribe to the idea that carbon dioxide is a pollutant, we respect your view. And even if that is true, regenerating the topsoil is still one of the easiest, most effective, cheapest, and safest ways of removing CO_2 from the atmosphere!

Ultimately do we even have any other option? How many of us can survive? Who knows! Let's switch to regenerative living and allow nature's laws to handle the population issue, as they always have.

Never forget that, despite the globalists' propaganda, you are *not* responsible for everyone! Your responsibility extends only to yourself and to your family and loved ones, to living an honest and decent life.

Yes, we *are* fundamentally good, we want to help each other, and to be free, sovereign wanderers and explorers on a clean, healthy, bountiful Earth. No, these things are not incompatible.

The vast majority of us, the 99.99% who are not psychopaths, share a similar point of view to that expressed in this epic monologue by Charlie Chaplin.

"I'm sorry, but I don't want to be an emperor. That's not my business. I don't want to rule or conquer anyone. I should like to help everyone - if possible - Jew, Gentile, black man, white. We all want to help one another. Human beings are like that. We want to live by each other's happiness - not by each other's misery. We don't want to hate and despise one another. In this world there is room for everyone. And the good earth is rich and can provide for everyone. The way of life can be free and beautiful, but we have lost the way.

Greed has poisoned men's souls, has barricaded the world with hate, has goose-stepped us into misery and bloodshed. We have developed speed, but we have shut ourselves in. Machinery that gives abundance has left us in want. Our knowledge has made us cynical. Our cleverness, hard and unkind. We think too much and feel too little. More than machinery we need humanity. More than cleverness we need kindness and gentleness. Without these qualities, life will be violent and all will be lost.

The aeroplane and the radio have brought us closer together. The very nature of these inventions cries out for the goodness in men - cries out for universal brotherhood - for the unity of us all. Even now my voice is reaching millions throughout the world - millions of despairing men, women, and little children - victims of a system that makes men torture and imprison innocent people.

To those who can hear me, I say - do not despair. The misery that is now upon us is but the passing of greed - the bitterness of men who fear the way of human progress. The hate of men will pass, and dictators die, and the power they took from the people will return to the people. And so long as men die, liberty will never perish...

Soldiers! don't give yourselves to brutes - men who despise you - enslave you - who regiment your lives - tell you what to do - what to think and what to feel! Who drill you - diet you - treat you like cattle, use you as cannon fodder. Don't give yourselves to these unnatural men - machine men with machine minds and machine hearts! You are not machines! You are not cattle! You are men! You have the love of humanity in your hearts! You don't hate! Only the unloved hate - the unloved and the unnatural! Soldiers! Don't fight for slavery! Fight for liberty!

In the 17th Chapter of St. Luke it is written: "the Kingdom of God is within man" - not one man nor a group of men, but in all men! In you! You, the people, have the power, the power to create machines, the power to create happiness! You, the people, have the power to make this life free and beautiful, to make this life a wonderful adventure.

Then - in the name of democracy - let us use that power - let us all unite. Let us fight for a new world - a decent world that will give men a chance to work - that will give youth a future and old age a security. By the promise of these things, brutes have risen to power. But they lie! They do not fulfill that promise. They never will!

Dictators free themselves but they enslave the people! Now let us fight to fulfil that promise! Let us fight to free the world - to do away with national barriers - to do away with greed, with hate and intolerance. Let us fight for a world of reason, a world where science and progress will lead to all men's happiness. Soldiers! in the name of democracy, let us all unite!" ~ Charlie Chaplin, The Great Dictator

If the idea that we can possibly survive without the leadership structure we have now seems bizarre or ridiculous, perhaps that is only because it is all you have known for your short life. The reality is that it is an extremely recent phenomenon.

Consider that we managed just fine for at least 95% of our existence living in harmony with nature's laws, having true leaders among us but without rulers or Owners. This new System is evidently not working, yet we are told we are not allowed to consider any kind of alternative, that the only answer is more globalization: global responsibility, money supply, food supply, and governance.

Or perhaps that is all just yet more bullshit, the final gasp for air of a dying System.

If you are feeling uncomfortable, angry, or scared right now, don't worry. Those feelings are totally normal, natural, and

243

appropriate. After all, the idea of disobedience being an evil has been drilled into us for our whole lives.

In fact we need to use that energy, because it has a creative power that we desperately need right now. Pain and fear often play a role in the cycle of death and rebirth.

It is now clear, *we* have to lead this. Any of us could be called to lead, and in different ways, from rediscovering true journalism or education, art or comedy, healing or religion, modeled on the true, eternal laws of nature, not the bullshit laws of Man's System. Perhaps we will discover a way back to paradise after all!

Listen for *your* unique calling. If you are being called to take a lead, lead in whatever way is right for you.

"In any one tribe there may be a hunting chief, work chief, dance chief, women's chief, age grade chief, and fishing chief. These leaders function only in specific contexts and for limited periods of time; usually, their primacy is based on capacity in the particular activity. It does not carry over into the round of daily life; and, almost everyone in the society is, at one time or another, in a 'chiefly' position." ~ Stanley Diamond, *In Search of the Primitive*

We do not need a change of leadership, at least not one that is stuck in the dysfunctional hierarchical model, with decisions made in remote corridors of power or in public-private partnership meetings at Davos. But we do need a new *definition* of leadership, to one that is truly transparent and accountable.

We can, and we must, build back better... And we're going to do it without Owners.

They are going to fight it all the way... but love conquers all. Nothing can stand in its way.

Let's stand for freedom, for choice, for true humanity... or at least the sovereign right to discover what that is for ourselves!

Remember, You are more powerful than they have allowed you to know. Why? Because you are part of the 99.99%, the greatest power in the world! If we stand together, nothing can stop us.

"Rise, like lions after slumber In unvanquishable number! Shake your chains to earth like dew Which in sleep had fallen on you: Ye are many, they are few!" ~ Percy Shelley

244

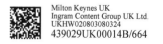
Milton Keynes UK
Ingram Content Group UK Ltd.
UKHW020803080324
439029UK00014B/664